Practical Applications in Dental Occlusion
Analog to Digital

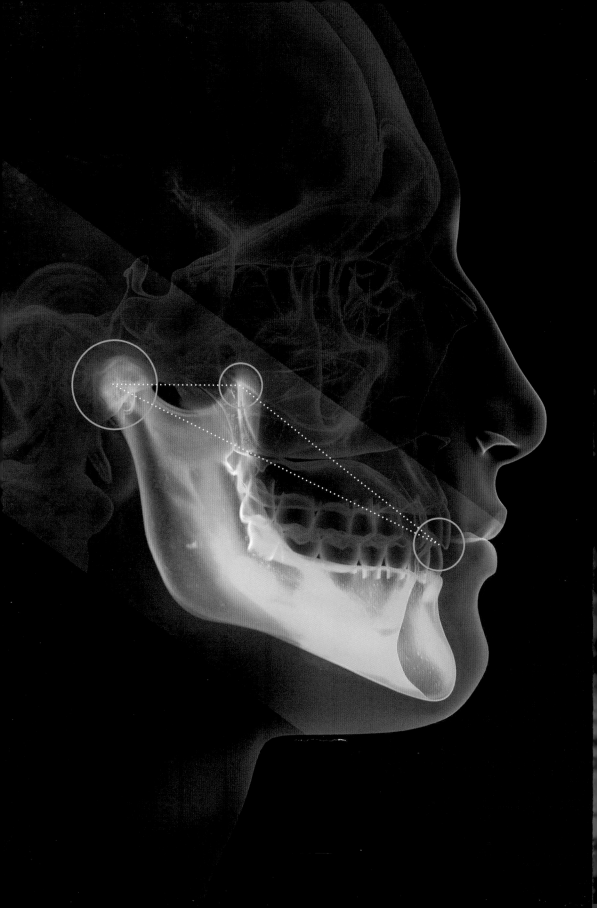

Practical Applications
in Dental Occlusion
Analog to Digital

Michael Radu, DDS, MS

Founder
Boca Institute for Dental Education
Boca Raton, Florida

With contributions from
Daniel Radu, DMD
Lee Culp, CDT

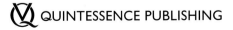
QUINTESSENCE PUBLISHING

Berlin | Chicago | Tokyo
Barcelona | London | Milan | Mexico City | Paris | Prague | Seoul | Warsaw
Beijing | Istanbul | Sao Paulo | Zagreb

One book, one tree: In support of reforestation worldwide and to address the climate crisis, for every book sold Quintessence Publishing will plant a tree (https://onetreeplanted.org/).

Library of Congress Cataloging-in-Publication Data

Names: Radu, Michael, 1955- author.
Title: Practical applications in dental occlusion : analog to digital /
  Michael Radu.
Description: Batavia IL : Quintessence Publishing, [2024] | Includes
  bibliographical references and index. | Summary: "Describes the two
  bites that are clinically possible--one where there is an existing
  occlusion and one where the occlusion must be newly constructed--and how
  to record and transfer this information to the lab for effective
  restorative treatment"-- Provided by publisher.
Identifiers: LCCN 2023056311 | ISBN 9781647241261 (paperback)
Subjects: MESH: Dental Occlusion
Classification: LCC RK523 | NLM WU 210 | DDC 617.6/43--dc23/eng/20240126
LC record available at https://lccn.loc.gov/2023056311

A CIP record for this book is available from the British Library.
ISBN: 978-1-64724-126-1

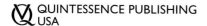 **QUINTESSENCE PUBLISHING**
USA

© 2024 Quintessence Publishing Co, Inc

Quintessence Publishing Co, Inc
411 N Raddant Rd
Batavia, IL 60510
www.quintessence-publishing.com

5 4 3 2 1

Editor: Leah Huffman
Design: Sue Zubek
Production: Sue Robinson

Printed in the USA

Contents

Foreword

Occlusion is one of the most confusing topics in dentistry. It has been taught over the last three-quarters of a century almost like religion. There is a "right way," which is the way the person teaching it describes it, and then the "wrong way"—anything other than what is being taught.

The good news is that the rigidity of some of the early approaches to occlusion have weakened. Research has shed light on the relationship of the occlusion to joints, muscles, and parafunctional activity. The challenge becomes how to now identify what is factual about occlusion and how that knowledge will influence patient care.

Dr Michael Radu has been practicing dentistry for over 40 years and has lived through the dilemmas created from the beliefs about occlusion. He is also a consummate student, who has exposed himself to varied beliefs by studying occlusion with several different individuals.

Dr Radu is also an excellent thinker. In this book, *Practical Applications in Dental Occlusion*, he recognizes that there are many facets to understanding and working with occlusion. It is, as he states, "a multifactorial topic."

His goals for the reader are to make occlusion practical and manageable, understanding that an appropriate occlusal therapy for some patients is not applicable to all patients. He accomplishes this masterfully by walking the reader through each facet of thinking about occlusion and then by evaluating how that thought process would alter the clinical treatment of the occlusion.

Along with practical language, the book contains illustrations that clarify the concepts being written about to make it easier for the reader to visualize what is being discussed, be they the relationship of the occlusion to the joints or the relationship between the teeth themselves in the different positions of the maxilla and mandible.

I am confident that if you read this book and allow yourself time to analyze what Dr Radu is describing, your understanding of occlusion will increase significantly, as will your competence and confidence in analyzing and managing occlusion for your patients.

Frank Spear, DDS, MSD
Founder, Spear Education
Scottsdale, Arizona

Affiliate Professor
University of Washington School of Dentistry
Seattle, Washington

Preface

Occlusion is often boiled down to the "tap, tap, and grind" of articulating paper marks we perform daily as practicing dentists. Our appointments each day are littered with fillings, single crowns, bridges, or more extensive fixed prosthodontics work. And for 90% of those appointments, we are able to ignore occlusion entirely until it's time to get out the articulating paper at the end of the appointment. Tap, tap, and grind. Drill the red marks. "How does that feel?" Tap, tap, and grind. Drill the red marks. "Don't worry; you're still numb and you'll get used to it." There is inherent adaptability in the stomatognathic system, which helps us even when we don't quite understand how to perfect the occlusion.

After all, 90% of the time, we can reduce the concept of occlusion into a consideration of the patient's current bite. We just have to adapt our treatment to that. But for the other 10% of the time, this approach will get us into big trouble. Sometimes the patient's current bite won't let us complete our treatment, at least not successfully in the long term. But if you don't know how to set up occlusion outside the patient's existing bite, what are you supposed to do?

Unfortunately, "occlusion equals confusion" is the catchphrase frequently repeated among dental students, and that attitude carries over into clinical practice. But occlusion doesn't have to be confusing. Not really. Not if you're taught how to understand and manipulate it. And that's where this book comes in—to teach you a simplified concept of occlusion that can help you perform predictable and successful treatment and avoid costly mistakes.

The book is divided into two parts:

- Part 1 outlines guiding principles and a simplified model of occlusion.
- Part 2 features specific situations you will come across as you diagnose, treatment plan, and treat your patients' cases.

A supplementary Notes section at the end adds a layer of theory and addresses the "yes, but there is more to it" concern.

My quest is to approach occlusion as a biologic system, uncover governing principles, and create order in a world of confusion. Occlusion doesn't have laws, models, and formulas like those found in mathematics and physics, but I draw from great thinkers like Pankey, Dawson, Spear, and Slavicek to provide you with simplified protocols you can adapt to your preferences. Let's ditch the indoctrination and controversy that plague our profession and focus on what we can achieve when we think well.

Patients come to us for many reasons. Sometimes it's clear what is needed, like a filling, while other times there is pain that we need to figure out and manage—or everything is broken down. Sometimes patients just want their teeth to look different. In all of these scenarios, we need to decide whether to keep the existing bite—the status quo—or change it. Most of the time we can help our patients without changing the bite. Sometimes we should change it, but we choose not to because it seems easier. And sometimes it is clear we need to change it. But do we let the patient determine the maxillomandibular position (ie, show us where they feel comfortable), or do we apply scientific principles to find the physiologic maxillomandibular relationship? At the end of the day, we need to answer three questions:

1. Do we keep or change the bite?
2. How do we change it if we need to?
3. How do we record the new maxillomandibular position for the lab?

This book will empower you to answer all these questions, every time. After reading this book, you will understand occlusion techniques using analog and digital workflows, including the following concepts:

• How to analyze occlusion
• How to decide to keep the existing bite or change it
• How to find the physiologic mandibular position when you need a new one
• How to record the new mandibular position for the lab
• How to integrate occlusion into your treatment plans

I hope this book helps to clear the muddy waters of occlusion and leaves you feeling confident and emboldened to treat your patients.

Acknowledgments

*"A man will turn over half a
library to make one book."*
– Samuel Johnson

It is my pleasure to express my deepest appreciation to those who helped me craft this book.

The first to mention is Leah Huffman, the editorial director at Quintessence Publishing. Leah was the smart and tough developmental editor who worked hard through multiple drafts to sharpen my messages. Thanks to her superb editorial instinct and clear vision, this is a much better book than it would have been otherwise. I owe her a ton of gratitude.

This book is also a result of having great mentors, such as Klaus Pfeiffle, Peter Dawson, and Frank Spear, to whom I owe most of what I know.

The book would have remained a perpetual project without Michael Noczinski and Gary Holland. Michael is my German master dental technician and partner in occlusion. We worked together for about 30 years, even after I crossed the pond. For years, he told me to stop talking about occlusion and just "write the book already." My dear friend Gary Holland, a successful businessman and fine intellectual, nudged me with his soft approach to commit to write what I was explaining to him and others about occlusion.

Lee Culp, my other incredible laboratory artist, was instrumental in developing my digital workflows.

My friends from the Scientific Investigation Committee of the American Equilibration Society deserve a big thank you. Our debates opened new perspectives and developed my thinking. Thank you Warren Jesek, Jette Holbrook, Jack Marincel, Scott Alman, and Keith Kinderknecht.

My colleagues in the Prosthodontics Department at Nova Southeastern University College of Dental Medicine shaped my knowledge and helped me meet and teach many students eager to learn why occlusion doesn't have to equal confusion.

Thank you to my closest dentist friends who read parts of the manuscript and helped me understand what wasn't clear enough and needed improvement: Irina Dragan, Radu Dogarescu, Titel Sufana, Anca Ralsen, and Marius Catiche.

A special thank you to Flavius Toma and Mircea Marandici, my engineer and scientist friends who verified my physics and the general principles guiding occlusion. Mircea deserves a very special thank you for co-authoring my article on the math of centric relation and distilling my intuitions into a simple formula. Our conversations are a source of inspiration, and it is amazing how much I learned from a non-dentist about occlusion.

My son Daniel is the one I have to thank the most for his contribution to this book. Our daily conversations, his deep and inquisitive thinking and skills in all things digital, and his help in refining my ideas over the years we worked side by side all helped shape this book. When we started to work together 8 years ago, he was the new dentist I was tailoring my writing for. He convinced me that besides knowledge, a dentist needs protocols. Later, my daughter-in-law Kristina became the new young dentist who showed me even more ways I would need to refine my message, and I thank her for her help.

Another group I have to thank are my patients and the incredible staff members of my dental practice—Tina, Laura, Jessica, Sharon, and Kim— my "work family." My growth as a dentist would have been stunted without their tolerance for my incessant desire to improve dentistry and try new techniques even when it meant extra work. They endured my passionate monologues and recurring frustrations with the status quo and heard me say the same thing a thousand times, with ever-so-slight differences along the way. Those differences are what refined my messaging and led to this book and its simplification of concepts.

Last but not least, I owe a lot to my family. My wife, Magda, and my sons, Michael and Daniel, have supported me and given me strength, even when that meant being away from them more than I liked. I have to thank Magda for allowing me to toil away for hours on end, both at work and at home, all to pursue my professional ambitions. She was always a bastion of strength in taking care of our sons and our home, all while having her own career.

This book is a work of love for my profession, patients, colleagues, students, and family. To all I owe my heartfelt gratitude.

About the Author

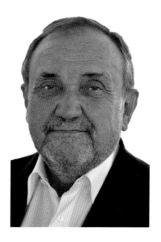

Michael Radu, DDS, MS, is a dentist who has practiced for over 40 years in three different countries across two continents. He believes strongly that his work is to help dentists with occlusion in their practice, so he lectures and educates his fellow dentists every chance he gets. He believes in science above all, which is why occlusion lies so close to his heart and why this book relies so heavily on the laws of physics. After all, Einstein explained how his relativity theory came from big scientific postulates, not from experiments, which may be biased, flawed, or misinterpreted.[1] Michael Radu also believes in the power of mentorship and the importance of sharing ideas to achieve new levels of understanding. Beginning with his physics professor in college and stretching to Klaus Pfeiffle and Michael Noczinski in Germany, Peter Dawson and Frank Spear in the United States, and the coterie of dentists at the American Equilibration Society, the support and positive challenges he was given have shaped his scientific approach to occlusion. In his eyes, the simplest, most irrefutable evidence is mathematics. When we think in terms of stability, vector of force, angles, and alike, we are less prone to make mistakes. Dentists will always prefer to work in the existing occlusion because no changes seem safer than the alternative, but Michael Radu challenges this notion and implores his colleagues to understand the scientific principles underlying the concept of occlusion so they can better care for their patients.

1. Einstein A. Induction and Deduction in Physics. Berliner Tageblatt. December 25, 1919.

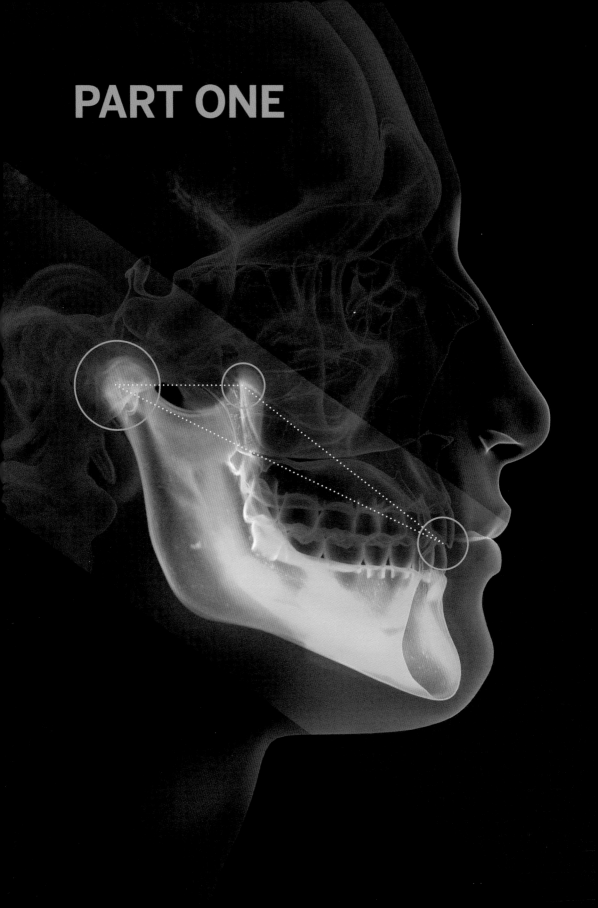

PART ONE

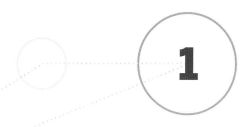

Why Do We Need Occlusion?

O cclusion seems complicated because it is a system with multiple parts, and our brains struggle to conceptualize and understand complex systems. As scientists, we want to understand the big picture of the whole concept, but as practicing dentists we need to figure out the details and identify an algorithm of steps to follow. This tension between the big picture and the details reflects how the right and left sides of our brain function,[1] and solutions to particular problems are only found when we get both sides working and integrate the details back into the big picture.

Occlusion: A Multifactorial Topic

Occlusion is a complex concept influenced by many problematic factors, as illustrated in Fig 1-1 and described in the following sections. This book acknowledges the problems and offers real solutions.

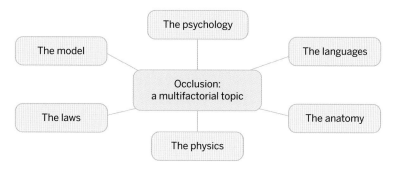

Fig 1-1 Mind map of occlusion.

The psychology of occlusion

PROBLEM: Our minds drive our behavior; essentially we become what we think about.[2] We fear the unknown, and occlusion is one of those topics dentists struggle to grasp fully. We learn about it in dental school, but we're still hazy on it when we graduate, and we're able to avoid it in practice by following certain rules: *(1)* don't change it; *(2)* if it's not broken, don't fix it; and *(3)* the patient will get used to it. But sometimes we actually do need to change it, we have to fix it before it breaks further, and some patients don't get used to it.

SOLUTION: This book presents protocols to combat the fear of the unknown.

The languages of occlusion

PROBLEM: Occlusion means different things to different fields of dentistry. In restorative and prosthetic dentistry, we change the tabletops of teeth to make them fit precisely together. In orthodontics, we move teeth to make them fit together, with some settling and adaptation. In maxillo-facial surgery, we move jaws and alter joints to make the teeth fit again, often with some orthodontics or restorative dentistry along the way. In operative dentistry, we keep the existing occlusion and make sure that we don't change it inadvertently. In periodontics, we usually keep the existing occlusion or perfect it to reduce the forces applied to certain teeth. In orofacial pain, we try to alter the occlusal patterns using an oral appliance.

Our terminology is at times a problem. Some terms are the same, some are different, some terms mean different things to different specialties, and some terms are dated but still being used in one specialty but not another. We speak different languages, and sometimes we need an interpreter.

SOLUTION: This book simplifies the terminology and seeks common denominators (see Note B).

The anatomy of occlusion

PROBLEM: Occlusion is a structured system with its own anatomy and internal workings. We need to understand how the system works to identify practical workflows for adjusting or recreating a patient's bite, but oftentimes this understanding is lacking. When we realize that occlusion is a structured system with commonalities and differences in individuals, we can better manage our clinical cases.

SOLUTION: This book shows how the system works and how to use it in practice.

The physics of occlusion

PROBLEM: We went to school to become doctors of dentistry. As such, we had to learn about the anatomy, biology, and neurophysiology of the human body, particularly the stomatognathic system. Once we had the scientific knowledge down, we had to learn how to use our hands to accomplish the fabrication and procedural work of dentistry. But dentistry is more than life sciences and art. As much as we want to solve medical issues for our patients, we need to acknowledge that biomechanics and physics have a huge role to play in our patient's mouths, especially when it comes to occlusion. And many of us did not become dentists to practice physics, so we have to learn it.

SOLUTION: This book presents a formula for occlusion that simplifies, quantifies, and creates a model to aid understanding of complex issues.

The laws of occlusion

PROBLEM: Occlusion has general laws and rules such as stability and adaptability, and the laws of physics also come into play when discussing occlusion. We need to work within these laws and stop trying to explain things superficially. For example, "the patient cannot tolerate a change in occlusion because of the personal stress" is an opinion, not a fact based on any scientific laws. A good occlusion must be stable—that is, it must be able to withstand the forces it is subjected to. We should never assume stability, but we often do.

SOLUTION: This book explains the laws of occlusion responsible for success in treatment and discusses the factors that influence stability. It presents checklists and protocols to ensure practical application of these principles.

The model of occlusion

PROBLEM: Any concept or system, no matter how complex, becomes more clear and understandable when we have a model to visualize it. Occlusion can be visualized as several models: a horizontal door, a tripod, a multilegged chair, or a mathematical formula containing its defining parts. But everyone thinks differently and processes information differently, so you need to find a model that works for you.

SOLUTION: This book presents all these models and suggests a few thought experiments to guide the reader in understanding.

Why Do We Need to Understand Occlusion?

There are three main reasons why we need to understand occlusion[3] (see Note A):

1. To decide which occlusion we should work in
2. To record it for the laboratory
3. To manage all the forces at play

First, we need to decide if we can work in the patient's existing occlusion or if we need to change it. In some cases there is no occlusion at all and we need to decide how to create one.

Second, we need to record and transmit the clinical situation (the "bite") to the laboratory so they can accurately fabricate the prosthetic pieces.

Third, we need to manage the forces applied to the existing teeth or newly created restorations to ensure stability and longevity. Occlusion is all about forces applied to teeth and other structures, and excessive forces are a potential pathogenic factor. In designing or maintaining the existing occlusion, we cannot forget about germs and the role they play in dentistry. We always need to prevent the overgrowth of bacteria by facilitating adequate hygiene access. Daily dentistry is really a study in germs and forces.

What Dentists Really Need

As dentists, we want to be able to apply consistent techniques and know exactly what to do in all clinical situations (Fig 1-2). That starts with the occlusal examination, diagnosis, and treatment planning and continues with the recording of the occlusion for the lab. In many branches of medicine, protocols have become the norm. They do not constrain the clinician to a set sequence but rather remind the clinician of the steps to be taken. Checklists are especially helpful in this regard.[4–6] In this book, a protocol or technique is presented for

Note: In this book, a protocol or technique is presented for every aspect of occlusion a dentist is responsible for. Because we cannot easily measure if we got the right bite, we need to apply step-by-step protocols to achieve the desired result.

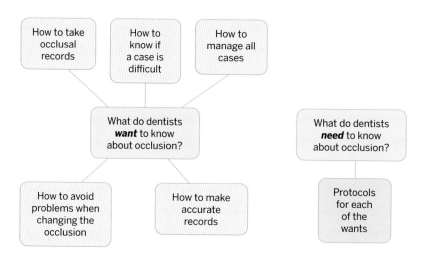

Fig 1-2 Mind map of the wants and needs of dentists regarding occlusion.

every aspect of occlusion a dentist is responsible for. These protocols help achieve consistency in the clinical steps to be taken and keep the focus on the desired goal—a healthy and stable bite. Because we cannot easily measure if we got the right bite, we need to apply step-by-step protocols to achieve the desired result.

Conclusion: An Analogy

I love to cook, and I love occlusion. Both are creative processes that rely on seeing the end result, following the recipe, making changes if needed, and fine tuning the result. Also, both get better with experience; the more you cook, the better your food tastes, and the more you practice occlusion, the better your patient outcomes. Experience means applying the process judiciously, not cutting corners, following the recipe but knowing when to change it slightly, and learning to correct mistakes to achieve the best end result possible.

References

1. McGilchrist I. The Master and His Emissary: The Divided Brain and the Making of the Western World. New Haven, CT: Yale University, 2009.
2. Allen J. As a Man Thinketh. Mount Vernon, NY: Peter Pauper, 1951.
3. Spear F. Fundamental occlusal therapy considerations. In: McNeill C (ed). Science and Practice of Occlusion. Chicago: Quintessence, 1997.
4. Gawande A. The Checklist Manifesto: How to Get Things Right. New York: Picador, 2009.
5. Brady W, de Souza K. The HEART score: A guide to its application in the emergency department. Turk J Emerg Med 2018;18:47–51.
6. Kavanagh BP, Nurok M. Standardized intensive care. Protocol misalignment and impact misattribution. Am J Respir Crit Care Med 2016;193:17–22.

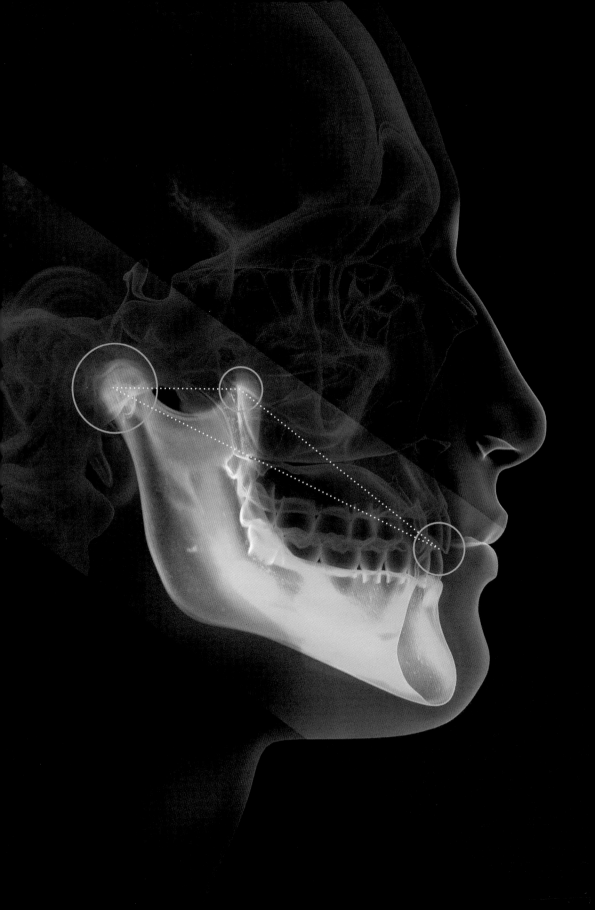

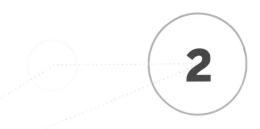

Practical Principles of Occlusion

Imagine you are a young person ready to learn how to drive a car. You come to class excited to get behind the wheel. But then the instructor walks in and starts teaching you everything about the rubber of the tires, the asphalt of the road, the motor under the hood, and the brake system. You want to learn how to drive the car. You don't care about the very important details of the rubber or the asphalt or the motor or the brakes.

With occlusion we have a similar situation. We learn in dental school everything about the anatomy and physiology of the stomatognathic system and its related structures, but we are never taught how to operate the vehicle. Occlusal textbooks abound on the details of the teeth, muscles, and joints (ie, the rubber and road in our car analogy), but what dentists want to know is how to manipulate the whole system in each clinical situation (ie, how to drive the car). I want to teach you how to drive.

Three Principles of Occlusion

To simplify and clarify the concept of occlusion, I suggest the following three principles, or self-evident truths. These are clinical and practical principles that relate to the big picture of occlusion.

Principle 1: Intercuspation is always associated with a mandibular position

Occlusion is many times equated to intercuspation (IC),[1] but occlusion is really a two-part system: one part IC and one part mandibular position (MP); note that the parts are not equal. As a mental model, think of the moving mandible and separate the parts: body, condyles, and teeth. The mandibular teeth are attached to a moving anatomical structure (the mandible) subject to the action of the masticatory muscles, so IC cannot be considered on its own. Because the mandible may have many positions without any IC, it helps to think of IC and MP as separate components, analyze them independently, and then relate them to one another (Fig 2-1).

MP is clearly related to the condylar position (CP). Most of the time, analysis of the MP is done at the condylar level and referred to as the CP in the fossa.[2,3] Some authors have even used the term "joint-based occlusion."[4]

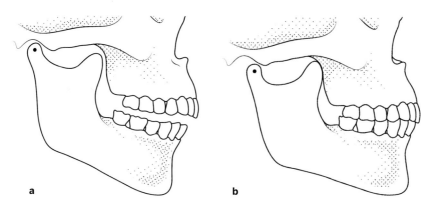

a   b

Fig 2-1 (a) MP with condyles seated in the fossae and no IC. (b) MP with condyles down the eminence and maximal IC.

Principle 2: The mandible is like a tripod

The mandible can be modeled as a tripod with two large legs in the back (the condyles) and many small ones (the teeth) working together as one in the front (Fig 2-2). The entire unit is seated by the force of the elevator muscles. The two condyles and the incisal point are far apart, and the vector force of the elevator muscles acts on the mandible how gravity acts on a tripod (Fig 2-3).

Fig 2-2 A depiction of an upside-down mandible as a tripod.

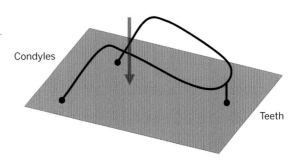

Fig 2-3 Drawing of the mandible, anterior teeth, and fossae as a reversed tripod.

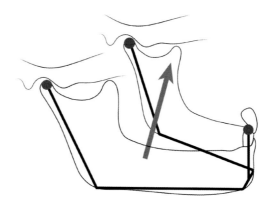

A table rests on the floor under the action of gravity; the mandible rests on fossae with slopes in the back (the joints) and uneven ground in the front (the cusps of teeth). Envisioning the mandible this way helps to create a visual and versatile model of occlusion. **Note:** This should not be confused with the "tripod of vertical support"—the three widely spaced occlusal contacts described by Freilich et al[5] and Squier[6]—or the "tripod advancement" described by Low et al.[7]

In the mandibular tripod as described by Woelfel[8] and Dawson,[9] two legs are the condyles and the third leg is the anterior teeth. With seated condyles and a single contact at the incisor level, the tripod is clearly stable. Okeson describes such a position as the musculoskeletally stable or stable orthopedic position.[10] A tripod cannot rock because it rests on a minimal number of supports. When the rest of the teeth intercuspate, there is a potential destabilizing effect. Like with a table, three legs ensure perfect stability, but four or more legs must have equal lengths to do the same. Under the force of the elevator muscles, with functional temporomandibular joints (TMJs), relaxed lateral pterygoid muscles, and no teeth interference, the mandible assumes the same seated CP repeatedly.[3]

Principle 3: A functional occlusion requires a stable MP

Stability is a general property of systems.[11] Like any natural system, occlusion seeks stability. This may be obtained through a stable IC and musculoskeletally stable joints.[12,13] In many clinical situations, a stable MP may be achieved through a stable IC (see Note D). In the absence of an IC (edentulous cases), or when we have to alter an existing one, the mandibular stability can be achieved by using a stable CP and an anterior reference point (see chapter 3).

A Mental Model of Dental Occlusion

A mental model is a simple, memorable visual representation to help conceptualize and make decisions about a complex system. Mental models are representations of reality in our mind. Peter Senge put it this way: "Mental models are deeply held internal images of how the world works, images that limit us to familiar ways of thinking and acting."[14] Mental models provide powerful tools to analyze the behavior of organizations and financial markets. A mental model of dental occlusion can do the same by eliminating the fuzziness of details and producing a simple mental picture containing only the main features.

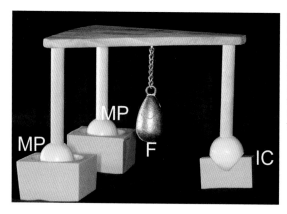

Fig 2-4 The mental model of dental occlusion. The model is a tripod with the two condyles seated in the fossae representing the MP and the IC as the third leg. The weight *(F)* represents the force of the elevator muscles.

This mental model of dental occlusion is not a biomechanical model that analyzes the forces and direction of movement of the parts involved in the system. Instead it provides a clear mental representation of how the mandible, muscles, and teeth work together. The opportunity to display the component elements helps you to better envision and understand how the system works (Fig 2-4). The tripod finds a stable position between the two condyles in the fossae and the intercuspal position, under the action of the masticatory muscles.

References

1. Angle EM. Classification of malocclusion. Dental Cosmos 1899;41:248–264,350–357.
2. Dawson PE. A classification system for occlusions. J Prosthet Dent 1996;75:60–66.
3. Radu M, Marandici M, Hottel TL. The effect of clenching on mandibular position: A vector analysis model. J Prosthet Dent 2004;91:171–179.
4. Piper Education & Research Center. Joint-based occlusion course. https://pipererc.azurewebsites.net/. Accessed 27 December 2022.
5. Freilich MA, Altieri JV, Wahle JJ. Principles for selecting interocclusal records for articulation of dentate and partially dentate casts. J Prosthet Dent 1992;68:361–367.
6. Squier R. Jaw relation records for fixed prosthodontics. Dent Clin North Am 2004;48:471–486.
7. Low L, Moore TE, Austin KR, et al. Mandibular "tripod" advancement of a Class II division 2 deepbite malocclusion. Am J Orthod Dentofacial Orthop 2010;137:285–292.
8. Woelfel JB. New device for accurately recording centric relation. J Prosthet Dent 1986;56:716–727.
9. Dawson PE. Functional Occlusion: From TMJ to Smile Design. St Louis: Mosby Elsevier, 2007.
10. Okeson JP. Management of Temporomandibular Disorders and Occlusion, ed 8. St Louis: Mosby Elsevier, 2020.
11. The Glossary of Prosthodontic Terms: Ninth Edition. J Prosthet Dent 2017;117(5S):e1–e105.
12. Zonnenberg AJJ. A Data-Supported Reference Position of the Intermaxillary Relationship [thesis]. Utrecht, Netherlands: Utrecht University, 2014.
13. McNeill C. Fundamental treatment goals. In: McNeill C (ed). Science and Practice of Occlusion. Chicago: Quintessence, 1997:309–311.
14. Senge PM. The Fifth Discipline: The Art and Practice of the Learning Organization. New York: Doubleday, 1990.

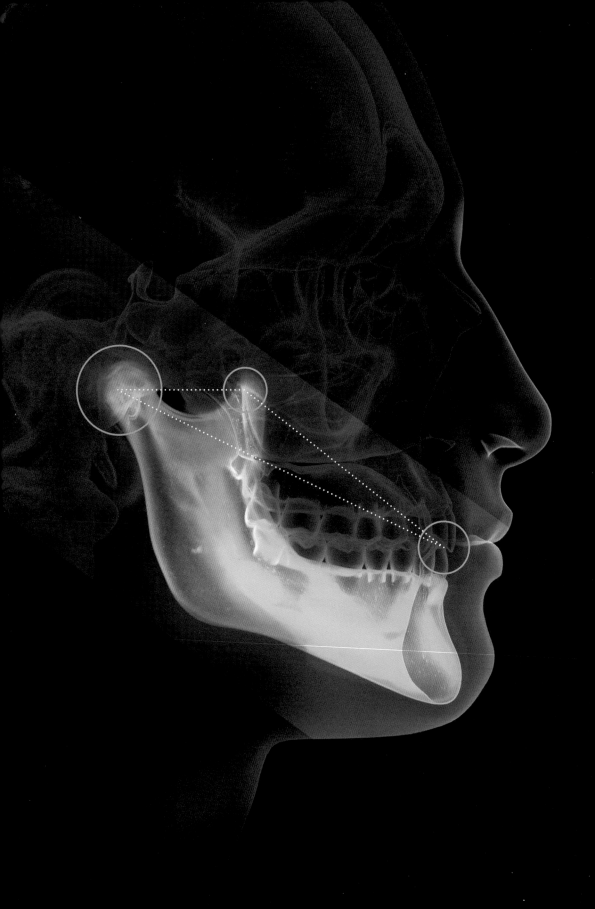

The Occlusion Formula

As introduced in chapter 2, occlusion is a system with multiple components. Besides intercuspation (IC, also known as *intercuspal position* or *maximal intercuspal position [MIP][1]*), the mandibular position (MP) also plays an important role. Because the maxilla is affixed to the skull, the mandible is the only moving part of the system. Thus, we are going to envision the mandible, in its entirety, as the main character in our story of occlusion. The mandibular teeth are affixed to the mandible, which must travel in order to acquire an IC. Therefore, every occlusion involves an MP associated with a given IC (Fig 3-1; see also Fig 2-1).

An analogy: Consider Einstein's space-time concept in which any object's position in space has an associated time. Just like there is no space without time, there is no IC without an MP.

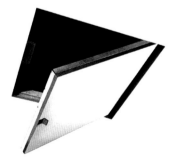

Fig 3-1 The mandible is like an attic door. The condyles are at the hinges of the door, which allows an infinite number of positions from open to closed. The edges of the door (ie, the teeth) can come into contact with the ceiling (ie, the maxilla) or remain out of IC. Being affixed to the mobile mandible, the mandibular teeth guide the mandible to a certain position in space when the hinge is closed. This is called the *mandibular position* and is an important part of the occlusion. The mandibular position is not readily visible, but it is always present.

We can summarize this with words as well as a formula to help create a simple model for understanding:

> **Occlusion is an intercuspated mandibular position.**
>
> $$O = IC + MP$$

(where the + represents an "and" instead of mathematical addition)

It is helpful to express complex systems and ideas in mathematical or logical equations.[2] This creates a simple model of the system.

The Role of Mandibular Position in Occlusion

To better define and understand the clinical implications of this functional relationship, we must further analyze the MP. Using mathematical concepts, the position in space of any rigid object is defined by three noncollinear points (not on one line). The anatomical shape of the mandible lends itself to good space definition because each condyle can be one of these points, while the midline incisal point can be the third. Together these points make the tripod discussed in chapter 2 (see Fig 2-3). In dentistry, we can define the position of the condyles in their respective fossae as the condylar position (CP) and the midline incisor point as the anterior reference point (ARP).[3,4]

VDO and ARP: The vertical dimension of occlusion (VDO) can be expressed as the position of the mandibular incisal point in relation to the fixed maxillary incisors. In other words, the VDO is how far away the moving mandible is from the fixed maxilla. It can be visualized as the mandibular incisal point in space.

If the MP is defined by the position of the condyles in the fossae (CP) and the mandibular ARP, we can express that mathematically as $MP = CP + ARP$ (Fig 3-2). Substituting this variable in

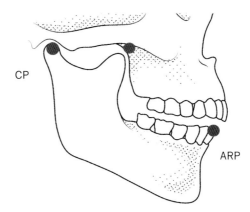

Fig 3-2 MP comprises CP and ARP.

CP

ARP

our previous formula, we have a new, more detailed formula for dental occlusion:

$$O = IC + CP + ARP$$

This formula separates occlusion into its base components, or the three variables we are always working with: IC, CP, and ARP. To clarify, this formula dictates the static occlusion, or the end position of the mandibular teeth in relation to the maxillary teeth. In other words, this is the occlusion when the teeth are intercuspated—when the patient bites.

However, we may also want to consider the trajectory of the closure—ie, the moving path of the mandible. The mandibular path in function is called the *envelope of function (EoF)*[5] and is part of the larger envelope of motion. The EoF is the portion of the envelope of motion when teeth are partially in contact. The dynamic MP in space is determined by the trajectory of the mandibular teeth and their interaction with the maxillary teeth in function and parafunction. This is referred to as *dynamic occlusion*.

Incorporating the EoF into our formula for occlusion, the complete static and dynamic occlusion formula becomes:

$$O = IC + CP + ARP + EoF$$

The recording of the EoF adds complexity and is a subject of analysis in chapter 10.

Practical Applications of the Occlusion Formula

While the condyles are hidden under the soft tissues, their position in space can be established and indirectly recorded in the mouth at tooth level using a substitute tripod. A tripod created by the incisal point (ARP) and the right and left second molars can be used as a substitute for the larger tripod of the ARP and right and left condyles (Fig 3-3). This allows an indirect recording (measurement) of CP and MP and eliminates the need for direct recordings, which are complicated because they require radiographic images of the condyles and complex analysis relating them to the dental arches. In other words, this substitute tripod makes a procedural criterion (finding the CP) measurable at the level of the dental arch. The second molars are used as the substitutes for the condyles because they are the most posterior points in the mouth, and the further apart the points are, the more accurate the MP is measured.

In the case of an *existing* IC, we record the MP using the teeth as landmarks. In the case of a *missing* IC (eg, fully edentulous cases or preparation of all teeth in one arch), we can create a tripod between an anterior stop (Fig 3-4) and the condyles as the posterior points.

The mandible is stabilized anteriorly using an obstacle adjusted at the desired ARP. The interocclusal registration is done intraorally in the posterior right and left areas using landmarks such as prepared teeth, occlusal rims (Fig 3-5), or recordings of the edentulous ridges (polyvinyl siloxane registration pastes or digital images). In these cases, the condyles are our invisible friends; they stabilize the mandible at the posterior end of the tripod and help us find and record the desired MP.

Important: The ARP is critical for MP stability and must be determined when the CP is established.

Fig 3-3 A smaller tripod using ARP and the position of the second molars (*purple*) can be used to substitute for the larger one (ARP and the condyles, *red*) and indirectly record CP and MP.

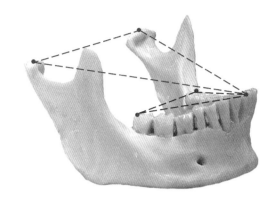

Fig 3-4 An anterior stop can be used to create a stable tripod using the condyles when there is no IC.

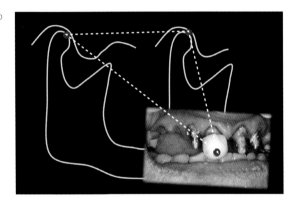

Fig 3-5 Three points on the mandibular occlusal rim are sufficient for a stable interarch record.

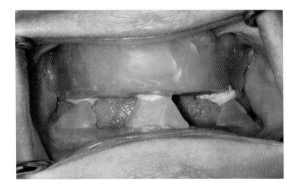

If we have an existing IC acceptable for treatment, we disregard the condyles and the ARP. In other words, we don't decide what MP (CP and ARP) to choose. Instead we make the decision to keep the MP acquired through the existing IC, and the simplified occlusion formula becomes $O = IC$.

Conclusion

The occlusion formula quantifies occlusion as a function of its parts and creates a mathematical model. It calls our attention to what we need to consider: the front end, the back end, the teeth, and the EoF.

In cases of an *existing* IC, every part of the occlusion is accepted as is. The system is adapted to that position (MP) and we want to keep it, because it ensures the stability needed. In cases of a *nonexisting* IC, every part of the occlusion is missing. We have to clinically establish CP, ARP, and EoF, and the laboratory establishes the new IC with the final prosthetic work, which we will insert in the patient's mouth. The system has no stability and is subject to many variables: muscle tone, head posture, operator's intervention, recording medium state, randomness. The clinician is responsible for ensuring a new MP stability to avoid the influence of the above variables. We cannot hope that a new random MP will produce a system stable enough to work within the patient's adaptive capability. After all, adaptation takes a long time to work.

References

1. McNeill C. Fundamental treatment goals. In: McNeill C (ed). Science and Practice of Occlusion. Chicago: Quintessence, 1997:309–311.
2. Nadella S, Shaw G, Nichols JT. Hit Refresh: The Quest to Rediscover Microsoft's Soul and Imagine a Better Future for Everyone. New York: Harper Business, 2019.
3. Nelson SJ (ed). Wheeler's Dental Anatomy, Physiology and Occlusion, ed 11. St Louis: Elsevier, 2020.
4. Wilkie N. The anterior point of reference. J Prosthet Dent 1979;41:488–496.

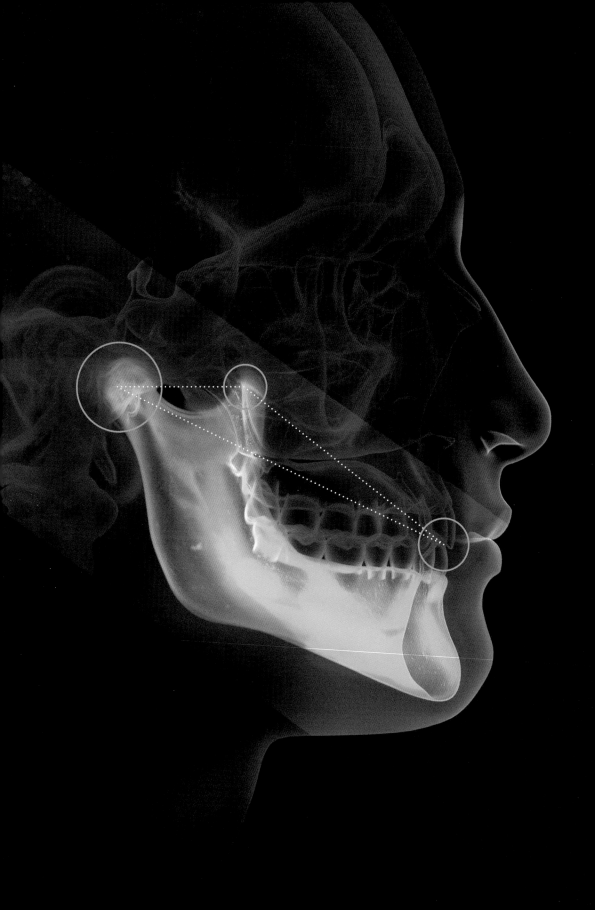

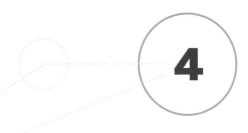

There Are Only Two Bites

An analysis of the occlusion formula (O = IC + MP) shows us that there are only two possible clinical situations: *(1)* when intercuspation (IC) exists and we can use that mandibular position (MP) for our treatment, and *(2)* when there is no IC or we need to change it. After all, MP is always present, but IC can exist or not.

In the majority of clinical situations, the mandibular teeth close onto the maxillary teeth in a functional way and no intervention is required from the clinician. Applying the occlusion formula (O = IC + MP), when we accept the MP created by the existing IC, the occlusion becomes synonymous with the IC: O = IC. This is the "no problem" bite. We don't want to alter it because it is a stable, habitual, good bite and allows us to complete the patient's necessary treatment in that position.

The difficulties and confusion begin to appear when we do not have an IC or we need to alter the existing one, as in the following scenarios:

1. The patient lost their maxillary or mandibular teeth, and the IC is missing.
2. We have performed a full-arch preparation on one or both arches, and the IC is missing.
3. The patient has spastic muscles and/or joint pain, and the MP is not in the correct place, so we decide to change it.
4. A patient with severe bruxism, worn dentition, and multiple missing teeth wants to have a better smile with longer teeth. In this case, we determine that while the existing IC and MP are functional, one or both aspects must be altered in order to achieve the patient's goals. This becomes scenario 2.

This is the "problem bite." The stability of the system has to be reestablished using a new MP, and an IC in harmony with that MP must be recreated. As clinicians, we must find a physiologic, orthopedically correct condylar (mandibular) position and record this position at tooth level so the laboratory can create the dental prostheses we request.

Essentially, there are only two bites, which are also two reference positions. One is created by the existing IC, and the other is created by the intervention of the clinician when the IC is missing.[1]

Bite One: The "No Problem Bite"

The existing IC, "no problem" bite is the standard clinical situation. We say we work "in what's there," hence the name *conformative occlusion*.[1] Most dentistry is performed in this "given bite," including operative dentistry, single or multiple crowns, partial dentures, and more. When there are enough teeth to guide the mandible in a definitive and stable IC, we can ignore the MP and consider the occlusion synonymous with the IC.

Bite Two: The "Problem Bite"

When there is no IC to use, we need to create a new occlusion, hence the name *reorganized occlusion*.[2] This is the "problem bite," because it requires the clinician to make some decisions. To record the bite in clinical situations when the IC is missing, we must find a stable, physiologic, orthopedically correct condylar position (CP) to provide stability at the posterior end of the mandible. Additionally, stability has to be provided to the front end, at the mandibular incisal point, using an obstacle between the arches.

We will discuss in-depth rationales for finding and recording both "bites" in Part 2. From the stability point of view, the existing bite has an acquired stability and the missing bite will need a constructed stability.

Conclusion

Describing the concept of occlusion as only two possible clinical situations helps to clarify the protocols/workflows of interocclusal registration. The criteria for determining which one to use are as follows:

- If possible and acceptable, use the existing occlusion (bite one).
- If no occlusion is present or the existing one does not allow for the restorative or functional goals, use a newly created occlusion (bite two).

The two occlusions are not two different standards of care—just two ways to achieve stability. The existing bite has an acquired stability that we accept as is, and the missing bite needs a newly constructed stability. In other words, existing bites are not substandard and created ones ideal; they are simply two different ways to achieve stability based on the presenting clinical situation.

References

1. McNeill C (ed). Science and Practice of Occlusion. Chicago: Quintessence, 1997.
2. Wiskott HW. Fixed Prosthodontics: Principles and Clinics. Berlin: Quintessence, 2011.

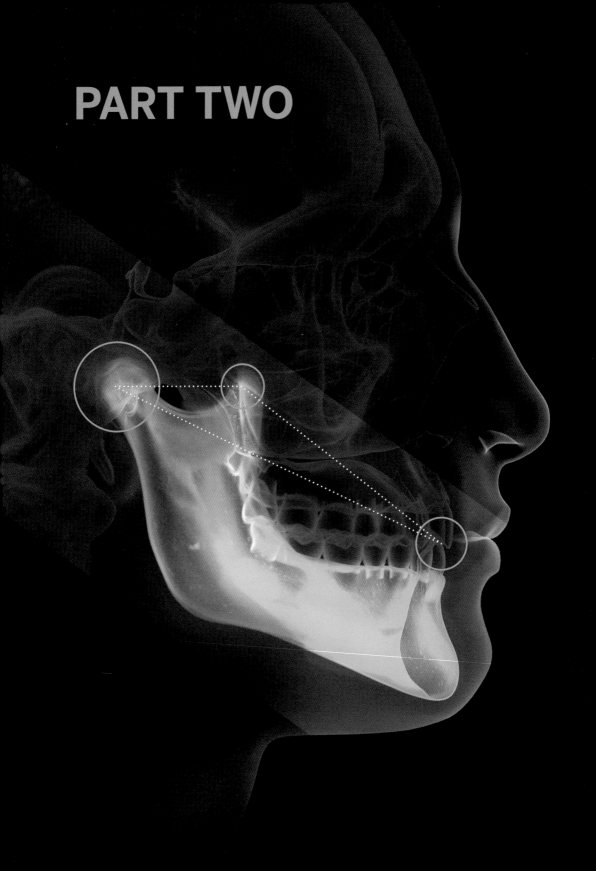

PART TWO

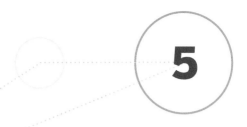

5

Clinical Techniques and Principles of Interocclusal Registrations

The theory behind occlusion is only useful if it can be applied clinically. As such, Part 2 of this book covers the clinical techniques for recording and deciphering occlusion, which are integral to the practice of dentistry:

1. **Techniques for examination and treatment planning:** Data gathering and planning is a preliminary technique and is a prerequisite for any treatment. Clinicians need a structured procedure (workflow) to examine the patient's occlusion and another to create a tentative treatment plan relating the patient's goals to the existing or future occlusion. These steps are vital, so a clear workflow is presented to use in all cases (see chapter 6).
2. **Techniques for interocclusal registration of an existing occlusion:** Most cases present with a stable occlusion that will need to be maintained. A structured workflow is still needed to minimize mistakes. Chapter 7 details the process for recording this static occlusion.
3. **Techniques for interocclusal registration for a new occlusion:** Recording occlusion where there is none is always challenging. Chapter 8 outlines the common denominator among these cases that unifies them as a category of interocclusal registrations. Again, this is a recording of static occlusion.

4. **Techniques for equilibration of the occlusion:** Besides recording the occlusion, dentists often intervene and adjust the patient's occlusion. Chapter 9 demonstrates the protocol for customizing occlusion for each individual patient.

5. **Techniques for recording the envelope of function (EoF):** Dynamic occlusion is just as important as static occlusion, and lab technicians depend on this information to create functional restorations. Unfortunately, clinicians often neglect to record the EoF. Chapter 10 therefore provides techniques to record the dynamic occlusion by capturing the EoF.

6. **Techniques for communicating with the laboratory:** For indirect restorations, communication with the lab is key. Chapter 11 presents a technique to ensure complete communication of all the data the lab needs to fabricate our restorations.

Interocclusal Registrations

Interocclusal registrations capture the spatial relationship between the maxillary teeth and the mandibular teeth. In reality, all interocclusal registrations are recordings of the mandibular position (MP) in relation to the maxilla, using teeth or substitutes (such as occlusal rims) as landmarks. Because the mandible is the only moving structure during the recording, its precise position must be captured. In this chapter, we discuss the stability of the mandible for the purpose of interocclusal registrations. A recordable position is one where the recorded structure is not moving—it is stable in space. To make sense of the techniques that follow in this book, the following principles of interocclusal registrations must be understood.

The mandible must be in a reference position

It is self-evident that we should not record a random position. We should record a reference position for the mandible that is reproducible and repeatable (see Note B). There are essentially two reference positions for the mandible: the maximal inter-cuspal position (MIP) and the stable condylar position (CP, sometimes called *centric relation*).

Asking the patient to "bite comfortably" in a recording medium will produce a random interocclusal registration.

The mandible must be stable at the time of recording

A moving body has a variety of positions, making it hard to record. The existing MIP is a reference position that is easy to accept and record because it gives stability to the mandible and establishes a CP and an anterior reference position.

In the case of a missing MIP, when we need to establish a new occlusion, we seek the other reference position—the stable CP. Because a body needs three points to define it, the condyles alone are not sufficient to stabilize or define the MP. A third point, the anterior reference point (ARP), is needed to stabilize the mandible (see chapter 3).

The recording relies on a three-legged landmark system

The MP recording is performed intraorally. Applying the principle that a tripod is the simplest stable system, when possible we choose three landmarks on the dentition or analogs of the dentition to form a triangle (see chapter 2).

The recording medium must not interfere with the MP

In the classic analog procedure, the recording medium is wax or poly-vinyl siloxane. However, wax may interfere with the MP and is prone to distortion. As a typical example, a wax bite rim used to record the MP in an edentulous case may be an obstacle to the closure of the mandible. Even the recording of a stable MIP may pose problems with any record-ing media.

In the digital workflow, on the other hand, the lack of recording medium results in more precise interocclusal registrations. The relative position of the two arches should be captured via intraoral scan to image the combined maxillary and mandibular position.

The transmission to the lab must be accurate and not prone to distortion

The digital workflow ensures easy and predictable transmission of interocclusal registrations to the lab. A significant advantage is that the technician does not have to manually articulate the models using the interocclusal registration.

Conclusion

All interocclusal registrations are recordings of the MP relative to the maxilla, and the mandible has to be immobilized (stable) for this static interocclusal registration. The trajectory of the mandible must also be captured for the dynamic interocclusal registration. Knowing the principles is a prerequisite to improving our techniques, not just performing these techniques often.

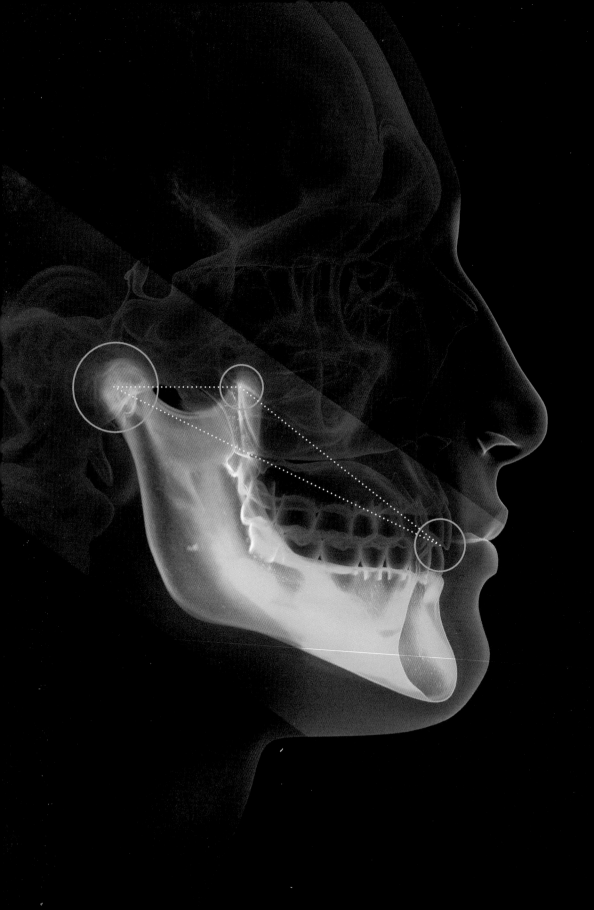

6

Techniques for Examination and Treatment Planning

The examination is the cornerstone of everything we do in our office. The examination leads to a diagnosis, which leads to a treatment plan, which leads to treatment (Fig 6-1). If there is no examination, then there is no treatment. If examination is incomplete, the treatment will be too. In fact, studies show that thorough examination, diagnosis, and treatment planning produces a more comprehensive treatment.[1] Comprehensive doesn't always mean large or complex—it just means that the patient is treated fully for their situation. In addition, taking time with the patient and being thorough with the examination creates trust and loyalty, which is rewarding in the long term.

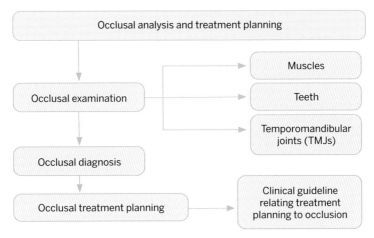

Fig 6-1 Mind map of examination, diagnosis, and treatment planning.

Note: The examination is always the starting point for building good rapport with the patient; do not underestimate its importance!

Examination

The initial patient exam has several components: history taking, cancer screening, structural evaluation (teeth and periodontium), functional evaluation (occlusion), and esthetic evaluation. This chapter addresses only the occlusal (functional) part of the exam, which is also the most often neglected portion. Keep in mind that the protocol outlined here for examination is appropriate for a cursory, or screening, exam. If significant signs or symptoms are revealed, the clinician should perform a comprehensive examination if proficient in that area or refer the patient to an appropriately trained clinician. Any treatment should be deferred until resolution of the problems. The examination, diagnosis, and treatment of temporomandibular joint (TMJ) disorders are beyond the scope of this book and can be found elsewhere.

The occlusal exam is central to comprehensive treatment planning. Many patients want to change the appearance of their smile. If we can help the patient understand that the function (occlusion) is the cause of their worn, chipped, or broken teeth, we become the expert they can trust.

A brief screening examination should be performed on all patients to quickly establish if we can treat the patient in the existing occlusion or if we need to address the occlusal problems first. In my 40 years of experience, I have seen three categories of patients: *(1)* patients with no significant muscle or joint problems (90%), *(2)* patients with moderate problems (10%), and *(3)* patients with severe problems (0.1%). In my career, I have referred fewer than 20 patients with significant joint problems to a TMJ surgeon (see Note F).

Nevertheless, the screening exam will tell you which category the patient fits into: the "no problem" category (90% of patients) or one of the "problem" categories (10%). These percentages are applicable for a general restorative dental practice, at least based on my experience.

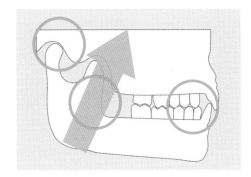

Fig 6-2 *(right)* Diagram of the components of occlusion: teeth, muscles, and joints.

Fig 6-3 *(below)* Occlusal examination form.

FUNCTION EXAM

History of complaints:		Muscles	Headaches	TMJ
Tender muscles		1–10	R	L
Masseter				
Anterior temporalis				
Middle temporalis				
Other				

Load joints		+	−
Prematurity:	Tooth # -		
Clicks:	Right	Lat. pole	Med. pole
	Left	Lat. pole	Med. pole
TMJ classification	- Piper:	1 2 3A 3B 4A 4B 5	
Occlusal classification	- Dawson:	1 2 2A 3 4	
Wear:	Anterior:	1 mm 2 mm 3 mm 4 mm	
	Posterior:	1 mm 2 mm 3 mm 4 mm	

Airway:	Acceptable	Deficient

These numbers will look very different in a practice dedicated to patients with temporomandibular disorders (TMDs). There may also be practices without "problem" patients due to the scope of practice or lack of attention given to functional problems.

Protocol for screening examination

Because occlusion is related to the muscles, condyles, and teeth, the occlusal examination must evaluate all these structures (Fig 6-2). Figure 6-3 shows the examination form to record occlusal data.

Palpation of muscles and joints

The screening exam begins with palpation of the muscles and joints.[2] This usually takes between 10 and 30 seconds, and the rationale is to uncover signs of overuse or latent damage to the anatomical structures.

Starting with the masseter muscles, use the index and middle fingers of both hands to palpate both sides of the face (Fig 6-4). Touch should be light at first, with rotating motion; if that elicits no discomfort, increase the pressure and ask the patient to report if they experience any discomfort or pain and to grade the discomfort on a scale of 0 to 10. This masseter palpation is a gauge of the possible occlusal-muscle problems. Most patients report a score of 0 or 1 to 3 discomfort, which indicates a "no problem" case. If the patient reports a score of 8 to 10, flinches, or pulls back from your touch, it may indicate a "problem" case; the patient may be experiencing muscle spasms created by occlusal issues or parafunctional habits (bruxism).

The same palpation approach is applied to the anterior and middle temporalis muscles and to the lateral aspect of the TMJs (Fig 6-5). Next, palpate the posterior aspect of each TMJ by inserting the pinky finger of each hand gently into the meatus (Fig 6-6). Ask the patient to open and close slowly to palpate a possible click. Note any audible clicks in the chart.

Performing this muscle and joint exam should indicate whether the patient falls into the "no problem" or "problem" category. To confirm the "no problem" categorization, go to the next step of the screening exam.

Joint loading

Joint loading usually takes 10 to 30 seconds, and the rationale is to establish if the joints can withstand load, which is a condition of a functional joint[3] (see Note H).

Fig 6-4 Palpation of the masseter muscles.

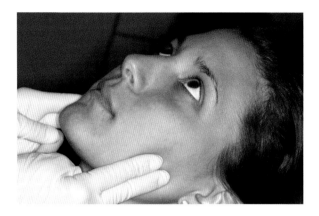

Fig 6-5 Palpation of the anterior temporalis muscles.

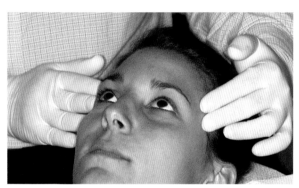

Fig 6-6 Palpation of the TMJs.

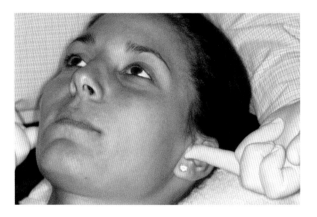

There are two tests that can be performed: *(1)* loading in the existing maximal intercuspation (MIP) and *(2)* loading in centric relation (CR) or seated condylar position (CP). (While "seated condylar position" is the technically preferred term, this text uses CR for clarity.)

Loading in the existing MIP is performed by asking the patient to "bite down on all teeth" and clench. If the patient experiences no discomfort in the joints, then they are probably in the "no problem" category. While this test is easy to perform, it is imperfect because the mandible is supported by the existing intercuspation (IC) and the muscles may not fully load the joints. Therefore, loading in CR must also be checked to prove that the joints can function in a fully seated CP under load (see Note E).

Loading in CR is performed using the bimanual manipulation technique (Fig 6-7) or a leaf gauge (Fig 6-8). With the leaf gauge technique, a sufficient number of leaves (usually about 20) are placed between the anterior teeth to ensure complete separation of the posterior teeth, and the patient is asked to move the teeth back and forth two to three times and then hold them in the back position and clench. This technique creates a tripod of support between the two condyles and the anterior obstacle (leaf gauge), with no support from teeth. If no discomfort is perceived, the joints are functional and we can proceed with treatment. If even a slight discomfort is elicited by clenching, we need to further investigate and heal the muscles and/or joints before proceeding with treatment.

A panoramic radiograph can be used to evaluate the condition of the condyles and establish if a more in-depth imaging examination (CBCT or MRI) is needed.

Interocclusal relationship of teeth

Evaluation of the interocclusal teeth relationship—or the bite—usually takes between 30 and 60 seconds, and the rationale is to uncover any signs of instability in the system. The instability may have two sources: the teeth themselves and the relationship between the MIP and CP (see Note B).

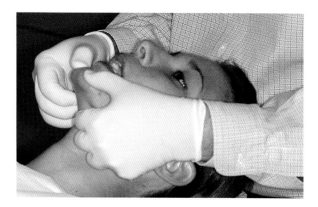

Fig 6-7 Bimanual manipulation technique used to load-test the function of the TMJs.

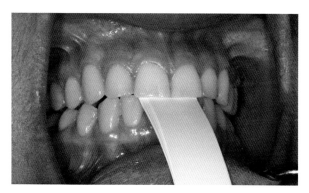

Fig 6-8 Leaf gauge technique to load-test the TMJs.

Teeth may have excessive wear or mobility, or there may be a reduced number of teeth, all of which are factors of potential instability. Any wear of anterior and posterior teeth is quantified and recorded in millimeters in the chart (eg, "mandibular incisors show 2–3 mm wear"). Tooth wear into dentin is a sign of instability, and because of the accelerated possible progression, it should be evaluated and presented to the patient. Any mobility of teeth is recorded on a scale of 1 to 3; it is a sign of instability and may indicate an occlusal overload. If there is a reduced number of teeth intercuspating, the stability of the mandible may be reduced, such as in an anterior open bite, so this too must be recorded and considered.

Relationship between MIP and CP

The relationship between the MIP and CP[2] is a complex and disputed issue (see Note E). We need to find out if there is a slide between CR and MIP. The question has to be asked during the examination, and the answer will follow us through the diagnosis, treatment planning, and treatment phases. To be clear, this text doesn't advocate eliminating all slides from CR to MIP, but we need to consider the existence of slides at the examination appointment. This is the time to find out if we have a slide, not later.

A coincidence of the CR and MIP (no slide) is considered a stable maxillomandibular relationship. In Dawson's classification of occlusion,[4] this situation is called Class I. In the general population, this is present in a very small number of cases (about 1%).[5] While it is desirable because it gives stability to the occlusion, it is impractical and unnecessary to make it the standard.[6]

To quantify a slide, you must establish the first point of contact in CR and then see the direction of deviation from the first contact to MIP. For example: "The first point of contact with condyles in CR is at #15, and the slide is 2 mm anteriorly and 1 mm to the left side." It is difficult to be that specific, but an effort to quantify the slide provides a record as to what the clinical impression was at the time of the exam. About 20% of patients have a shift greater than 2 mm, and most people have a shift between 0.5 and 2 mm.[5] When the shift is greater than 2 mm, there is a risk that the patient will lose the intercuspal position when the posterior teeth are prepared.

Mounted study models

Study models have historically been a great tool to document, evaluate, plan treatment, and communicate the state of the arches and the relationship between them. They are also a great point of debate: Should we make them for all patients or only for the ones needing extensive treatment? Should we mount them by hand articulation or in CR? Are

Fig 6-9 Analog study casts require a separate appointment and are harder to use as a communication tool with patients.

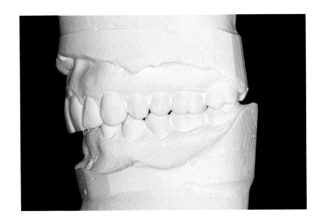

they worth the time and additional appointment needed for the patient? All of these issues are relevant with the analog workflow of taking impressions, pouring the casts, and mounting them in an articulator (Fig 6-9). However, the digital workflow eliminates many of the negatives and adds several benefits.

With the digital workflow, at the end of the clinical examination, the dentist or assistant can scan the maxillary and mandibular arches in about 2 minutes using an intraoral scanner. An interocclusal registration can be taken in MIP and/or in CR in about 1 minute. The digital models are available immediately, and the condition of the teeth can be discussed with the patient at the same appointment, including old restorations, cracks, fractures, wear, abfractions, color, crowding, missing teeth, gingival recessions, and the "bite" (Fig 6-10). The patient can easily understand the digital scans and even see the "bite" discrepancies.

Important: Do not skip any part of the occlusal examination. It is essential for the treatment planning.

In the 5 minutes it takes to perform the occlusion screening exam and capture digital scans and occlusal records, we have a complete picture of the function of the patient, with the structures visible in color and in function. Communication with the patient becomes easy and clear, and the needed treatment is almost obvious.

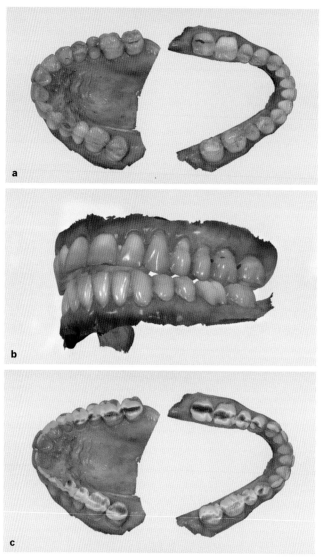

Fig 6-10 *(a to c)* Digital study casts (scans) are immediately available after scanning to show the patient the condition of their teeth, including how the teeth articulate with seated condyles and why the bite is unstable. The patient can also see the first point of contact *(in dark blue)* and visualize the space between the other teeth with the color gauge.

Fig 6-11 Treatment planning done while looking at the patient's smile: veneers needed on maxillary anterior six and incisal composites needed on mandibular anterior six.

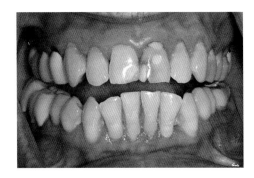

Diagnosis

Diagnosis is the determination of the nature of the disease or the process of finding the cause of the patient's signs and symptoms. A diagnosis regarding occlusion may read something like this: "Discrepancy between CR and MIP, with 2-mm slide, muscle tenderness on palpation, bilateral pole click, and 2 to 3 mm of wear of the anterior maxillary teeth." For patient communication, the same diagnosis should be worded differently: "Excessive tooth wear and muscle pain due to misalignment of the bite." The diagnosis is the conclusion of the examination and creates a correlation between the findings. It also allows us to have a prognosis.

Treatment Planning

There are books, courses, and mini-residencies dedicated to the topic of treatment planning. Treatment planning can be a complex process, but the occlusion planning can be systematic with the help of a clear protocol, as outlined in this section.

What to avoid

Clinicians often consider treatment planning to be a list of procedures they dictate to the assistant while looking at a set of radiographs or into a patient's mouth (Fig 6-11). However, there are at least two problems with this approach: First, the patient may want something very different than what the dentist has in mind, and second, the function of the stomatognathic system and the esthetics cannot be evaluated on radiographs or by simply looking at the teeth. In other words, treatment planning has to be done in three dimensions, considering the mandibular function.

Principles of treatment planning

Treatment planning must take into account the patient's objectives for treatment. The patient may have clear objectives when walking into the office, or the objectives may be developed at the examination and diagnosis appointment, when the dentist makes suggestions for treatment options. Whatever the case may be, the patient's wants and needs must be in agreement with the technical realities of the case. We may create a before and after projection with an imaging program (Fig 6-12), but we also need to make sure we can implement it in the mouth.

Treatment planning must also take into account the function, as well as the structure and esthetics. You cannot just give a patient esthetic restorations and hope for the best. If you place a full-coverage anterior restoration in a mouth that doesn't have the vertical dimension of occlusion (VDO) to accommodate it,[7,8] you will create a posterior open bite, unless more restorations for the posterior teeth will be made (Fig 6-13). By correcting the esthetics, you will have created functional problems for the patient. Keep in mind the occlusion formula: O = IC + CP + ARP. If you change the anterior reference point (ARP) by adjusting the VDO, then you will also change the occlusion.

Fig 6-12 Imaging software creates before and after views to show the patient potential smile improvements.

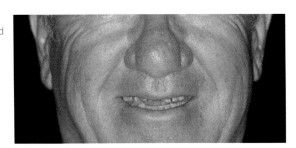

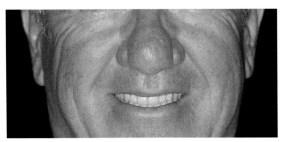

Fig 6-13 Diagram showing the need for complete arch restoration when the VDO has been increased to accommodate the anterior esthetic restorations.

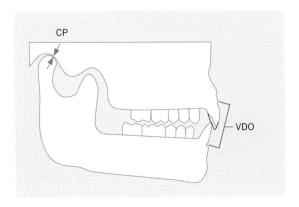

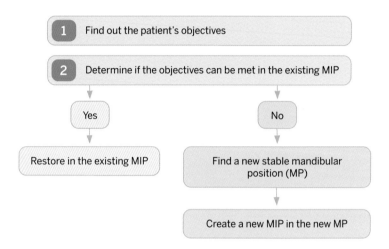

Fig 6-14 Clinical guideline relating treatment planning to occlusion.

Guideline relating treatment planning to occlusion

A broad definition of treatment planning is the process by which we understand and fulfill the patient's objectives (see Note C). For clarity and consistency, the process has to follow a set of guidelines (Fig 6-14):

1. Find out the patient's objectives and discuss their feasibility.
2. Evaluate if the treatment objectives can be achieved in the existing MIP or if a change in occlusion is needed.
3. If the existing MIP can be maintained, proceed with treatment in that mandibular position (MP).
4. If the MIP has to change or is not available, record a new MP with the condyles fully seated and the incisal point at the desired VDO (ARP).
5. Make a treatment plan to re-create the MIP in that MP, first as a mock-up (analog or digital).

Fig 6-15 The patient wants longer teeth and structural improvement.

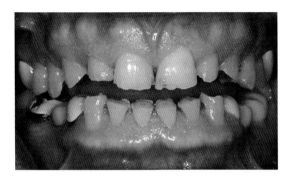

Clinical example

The first question in the guideline is: What are the patient's objectives? Does the patient want the smile restored or just a broken tooth repaired? This information is critical. As dentists, we must consider the patient's objectives and either limit the plan to that or make the case for a different plan. Sometimes what the patient wants is not feasible or more dentistry is needed to solve the problem. In the case presented in Fig 6-15, the patient wants to look better and protect the worn teeth from further damage.

The second question is: Can we do it in the present occlusion? In other words, can we keep the existing occlusion unchanged and achieve the patient's objective in that bite? There is plenty of treatment we can do in the given bite: fillings, single crowns, sometimes bridges, or even anterior cosmetic work. As a percentage of dental services offered, most practices perform around 90% of work in the existing occlusion. Daily routine work is done in the existing bite most of the time. For the patient in this clinical example, can we achieve his objectives of better esthetics and protection from further wear in the existing occlusion (Fig 6-16)? The answer is no; we have to open the VDO (changing the ARP), change the MP, and restore IC in the new MP (Fig 6-17).

Note: A good treatment plan is the one in the right MP. If you make beautiful restorations in the wrong MP, the treatment will not be successful because the patient cannot function.

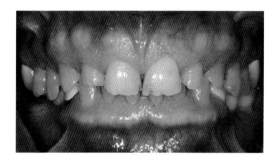

Fig 6-16 Can better esthetics be achieved in the existing occlusion? No, we need to increase the VDO.

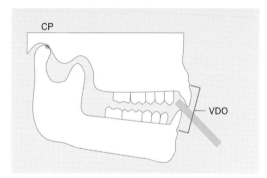

Fig 6-17 We establish a new MP, with the condyles fully seated, at the desired VDO, which creates a new ARP for our occlusion.

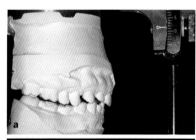
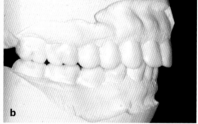
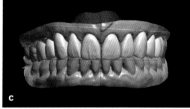

Fig 6-18 *(a and b)* Analog wax-up. A new MP is determined by the seated condyles in their fossae and the incisal point at the desired opening. *(c)* Digital wax-up.

The new MIP is recreated virtually first with a wax-up, made with either an analog or digital workflow (Fig 6-18). The clinical modalities available to re-create the MIP include equilibration, orthodontics, restorative dentistry, and maxillofacial surgery.

An analogy

In his bestselling book *The 7 Habits of Highly Effective People,*[9] Steven Covey highlights the principle of beginning with the end in mind. An example he gives is the difference between a manager and a leader. Management is doing things right, while leadership is doing the right thing. In the case of woodworkers cutting trees in a forest, the manager prepares the workers and the tools for efficiency to increase production. The leader, meanwhile, climbs the tallest tree, surveys the situation, and yells, "Wrong forest!"

In treatment planning with occlusion, sometimes we work hard toward making the teeth match in a perfect IC. But our first question should always be: Are we in the right MP?

Esthetic Dentistry and Occlusion

Esthetic dentistry has taken up a large portion of dentistry. After all, who wants to have ugly teeth? Students are taught in dental school about the principle of esthetic dentistry, and there are academies and societies dedicated to these concepts. There are esthetic norms and rules, and we have very clear guidelines regarding what makes a smile beautiful—norms for incisor position and shape, the smile line, the buccal corridor, and more. These features of the smile are analyzed mainly on photography, which is a 2D analysis. In the mouth of the patient, however, there are also functional issues to resolve, such as the movement of the mandible (and the mandibular teeth), and function happens in 3D. This discrepancy between esthetic evaluation and functional evaluation may create a conflict between where we want the teeth to be and where they should be from a functional point of view.

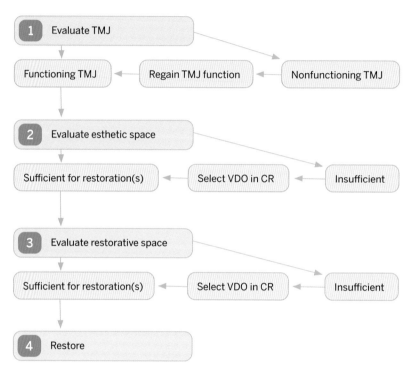

Fig 6-19 Decision tree for restorative cases.

Therefore, the esthetic analysis should have two parts: the smile design (2D on analog or digital photography) and the occlusal design (3D on analog or digital articulators). Esthetic dentistry is closely related to occlusion because altering teeth for esthetic purposes may interfere with the envelope of function (EoF). Also, esthetic dentistry has to be considered in the big picture of any restorative case. A decision tree to consider in all cases is presented in Fig 6-19, and Fig 6-20 presents a decision tree for when the MIP or VDO needs adjustment prior to restoration.

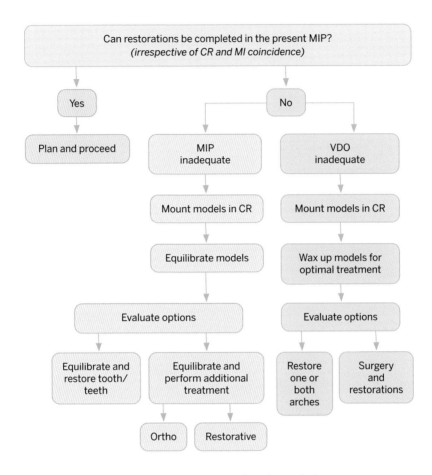

Fig 6-20 Decision tree for determining next steps based on occlusion.

Conclusion

The occlusal examination, diagnosis, and treatment planning are clinical techniques to be mastered as a prerequisite for treatment. To treatment plan, we must examine and diagnose first, and occlusion is an integral part of that planning. Box 6-1 lists some common questions regarding occlusal examination and diagnosis and their relevant answers.

Box 6-1	**Common questions about occlusion examination and diagnosis**

Q | **Why do I have to do a special occlusal exam? Is that not part of the general exam?**

Many times, dentists examine carefully for caries, periodontal disease, and missing teeth. The function of the stomatognathic system, which is the occlusion, may be neglected if the patient does not have specific complaints regarding it. Occlusion is not only an important pathogenic factor, but it also plays a crucial role in planning for any significant treatment.

Q | **What radiographs or tests are required to properly diagnose the TMJs and other related structures?**

In this chapter, we addressed only the screening examination for occlusal problems. TMJ imaging for complex cases of jaw joint problems is beyond the scope of this book and should be referred to a clinician with the requisite knowledge and experience to treat such cases.

Q | **How do I inform the patient about a click that I uncovered when I'm not very familiar with the pathology of the joints?**

If the patient is not aware of a click and you uncover it, it is beneficial to let them know. On one hand, it means that your treatment did not provoke the click; on the other, it brings up a discussion with the patient about the health of the TMJs. If indeed there are problems, you can refer the patient to a health care provider who treats such problems. The reality is that we, as dentists treating the stomatognathic system, should have a certain level of knowledge regarding the joints, at least enough to know when we can treat that patient and when we need to refer to a clinician proficient in this field.

References

1. ADA Report on Fees. https://ebusiness.ada.org/login/login.aspx?cpssource=https://www.ada.org/login?returnUrl=https://www.ada.org%2fresources%2fcareers%2fcompensation-as-an-employee-or-associate-dentist%26assetRedirect%3d%2f. Accessed 9 March 2023.
2. Okeson JP, Kazumi I. Orthodontic therapy and the temporomandibular disorder patient. In: Graber LW, Vanarsdall RL, Vig KWL (eds). Orthodontics: Current Principles and Techniques, ed 5. Elsevier, 2012:179–192.
3. Dawson PE. Functional Occlusion: From TMJ to Smile Design. Elsevier, 2007.
4. Dawson JP. A classification system for occlusions. J Prosthet Dent 1996;75:60–66.
5. Utt TW, Meyers CE Jr, Wierzba TF, Hondrum SO. A three-dimensional comparison of condylar position changes between centric relation and centric occlusion using the mandibular position indicator. Am J Orthod Dentofacial Orthop 1995;107:298–308.
6. Zonnenberg AJJ. A Data-Supported Reference Position of the Intermaxillary Relationship [thesis]. Utrecht, The Netherlands: Utrecht University, 2014.
7. Calamita M, Coachman C, Sesma N, Kois J. Occlusal vertical dimension: Treatment planning decisions and management considerations. Int J Esthet Dent 2019;14:166–181.
8. Goldstein G, Goodacre C, MacGregor K. Occlusal vertical dimension: Best evidence consensus statement. J Prosthodont 2021;30(S1):12–19.
9. Covey SR. The 7 Habits of Highly Effective People. New York: Free Press, 2004.

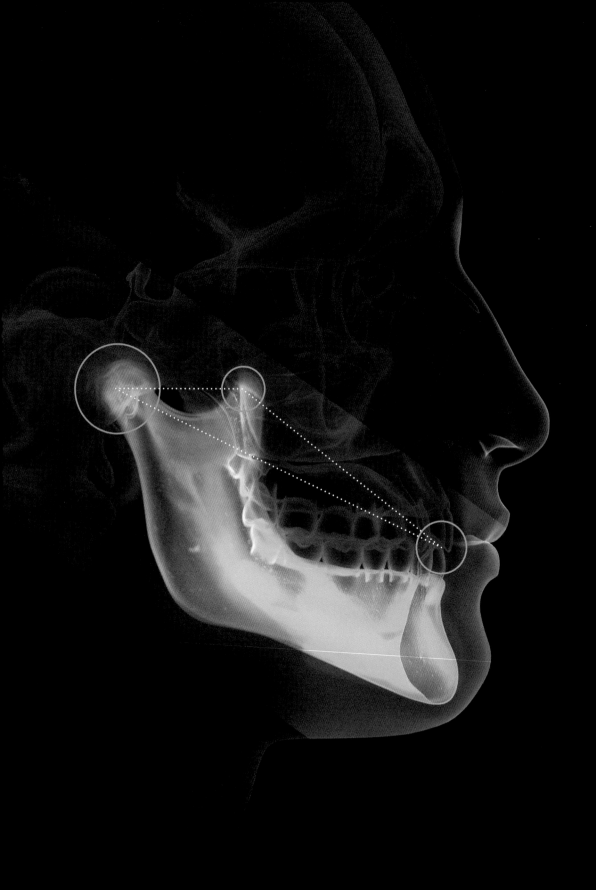

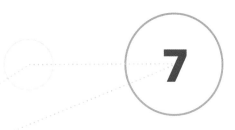

Techniques for Interocclusal Registration of an Existing Occlusion

With contributions from Daniel Radu, DMD

Recording the occlusion for the lab is a routine procedure in clinical practice. We ask the patient to "bite down" and interpose a recording medium between the arches, or we use digital scans and occlusal records to record the existing occlusion. This existing occlusion, or maximal intercuspation (MIP), is a reference position[1] also known as *conformative occlusion*.[2] This is the "no problem" bite, and the occlusion formula is simplified as O = IC.

This chapter presents the analog and digital workflows for interocclusal registrations for single-tooth crown preparation, multiple-tooth preparation with potential mandibular instability, terminal tooth position, and implant restoration within the existing MIP (Fig 7-1). The goal of any interocclusal registration is to accurately record the interocclusal relation and transmit it distortion-free to the lab, and this chapter will teach you how to accomplish that goal.

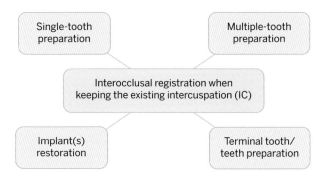

Fig 7-1 Mind map of interocclusal registrations of conformative occlusion.

Single-Tooth Preparation Interocclusal Registration

The patient in Fig 7-2 presented with a crack involving the buccal cusp of a maxillary premolar, and the decision was made to restore it with a full-coverage restoration. The restorative space was sufficient to accommodate the proposed restoration, so the existing occlusion could be maintained. Therefore, the condylar position (CP) and anterior reference point (ARP) of the occlusion formula could be disregarded, because occlusion equated to intercuspation (IC) only.

For interocclusal registration of single-tooth preparation, we need to give the lab the maxillomandibular relationship (MMR) record in the existing MIP. That means we must be careful not to *alter* the MIP in the process of recording it. The following sections therefore outline analog and digital protocols for interocclusal registration for single-tooth preparation in existing MIP (see Note B).

Note: The single-tooth preparation interocclusal registration also applies to multiple-tooth restorations in one arch where there are sufficient other teeth to provide stability to the mandible, for example as shown in the three–unit fixed partial denture preparation in Fig 7-3.

If the patient has healthy muscles and joints and the restorative space is sufficient, the author recommends proceeding with full-arch impressions or scans in order to give the lab the possibility of replicating the envelope of function (EoF). Partial impressions or scans are not sufficient to replicate the EoF, and the clinician may need to make extensive adjustments of the restoration intraorally.

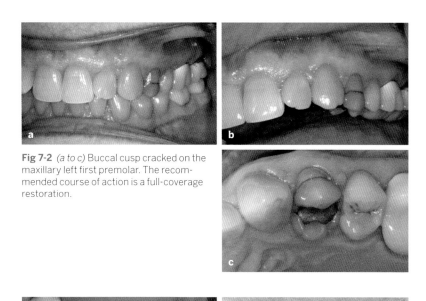

Fig 7-2 *(a to c)* Buccal cusp cracked on the maxillary left first premolar. The recommended course of action is a full-coverage restoration.

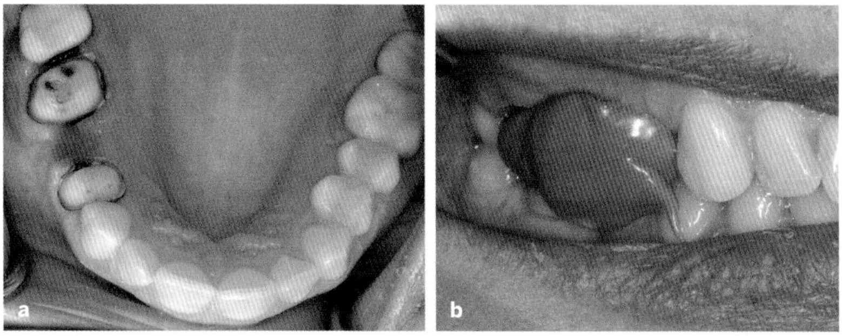

Fig 7-3 *(a and b)* Interocclusal registration of multiple prepared teeth for a three-unit fixed partial denture, with sufficient stability provided by the adjacent unprepared teeth.

Analog technique

1. Place polyvinyl siloxane (PVS) bite registration paste (Blue Mousse, Futar, etc) or wax in the prepared area, and ask the patient to bite on all teeth. Be sure to check that closure is complete, and wait until full setting of the paste or wax before proceeding.

2. The wafer of registration material, limited to the prepared area, is helpful in the articulation process. The wafer must be trimmed to the point of leaving only a few clear surfaces for articulation (Fig 7-4). If the registration material is placed in unprepared areas where there is minimal space, trimming will be difficult, and the result will be a questionable model position during articulation (Fig 7-5).

3. Pack and send the impressions and interocclusal registration to the lab.

4. The lab technician will articulate the models with the help of the PVS bite record and place them into an articulator (Fig 7-6). The process of articulation in the lab is a potential source of imprecision because of the many variables involved (models, occlusal record, human factors).

Fig 7-4 PVS occlusal record trimmed to allow precise seating of the models.

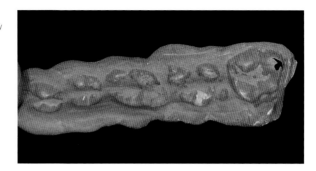

Fig 7-5 PVS occlusal record not trimmed, potentially leading to imprecise articulation.

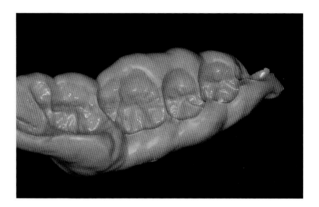

Fig 7-6 Laboratory articulation of models using a PVS occlusal record.

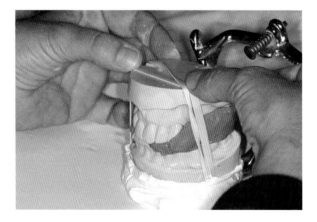

Digital technique

1. Place the head of the intraoral scanner (IOS) on the right side of the arches, record the interarch relationship, and then repeat the same on the left side (Figs 7-7a and 7-7b). The MMR record is a buccal scan of both arches. The IOS software creates the interocclusal registration in MIP by matching the digital casts of the arches to the buccal scan (Fig 7-7c).

2. Some IOSs allow recording of the mandibular movement as well, which can be used by the lab technician to design an occlusal surface in harmony with the mandibular movements (ie, it respects the EoF; Fig 7-8). An alternative technique is to make a prepreparation scan and use it to design the new restoration. This works when sufficient occlusal anatomy is available.

3. Upload the digital casts and occlusal record scans to the lab's CAD/CAM software. Pay attention to the "intersections" (Fig 7-9), which the scanning software can compensate for. Intersections are inter-mesh penetrations between opposing arch surfaces resulting in inaccurate MMR in the virtual casts.[3]

4. The lab technician will use the data for the digital design and fabrication of the prosthetic device.

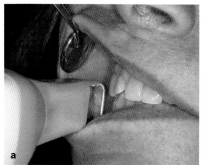
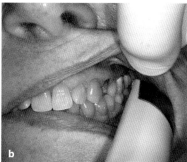

Fig 7-7 *(a and b)* The IOS is placed in the right and left buccal corridors while the patient closes in MIP. *(c)* The digital interocclusal registration in MIP *(in light blue)* matches the full-arch scans into an articulated set of digital casts to be placed in the virtual articulator.

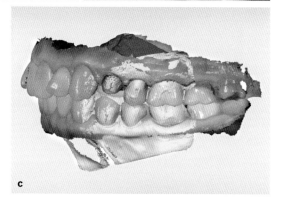

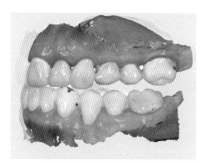

Fig 7-8 Mandibular movements recorded using the "patient-specific motion" function with the TRIOS (3Shape) IOS.

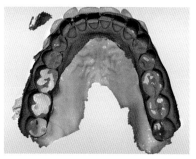

Fig 7-9 Digital occlusal records with so-called "intersections," where opposing teeth seem to collide in the molar area, especially on the right side.

Multiple-Tooth Preparation Interocclusal Registration

When preparing only one tooth, especially in an intercuspated position, the MMR stability is easy to maintain—it's the same as before the preparation. When more teeth are prepared and come out of contact (ie, lose their relationship with the opposing one), however, as shown in Fig 7-10, the less stable the MMR becomes and the more questionable the interocclusal registration becomes. This section uses preparation of the six maxillary anterior teeth as a representative example of multiple-tooth preparation interocclusal registration, as this is a common clinical scenario.

When the limited MIP on the posterior teeth still ensures stability, we can proceed with the registration. To prevent any inadvertent movements that could threaten the stability of the MMR, a composite resin stop is recommended in the area of the central incisors to further stabilize the MMR:

1. Place a composite resin stop on the palatal surface of one or both of the maxillary central incisors (Fig 7-11). Alternatively, a composite stop can be placed on the incisal edge of the mandibular central incisors. Do not etch; just apply the bonding agent and cure prior to fitting the composite resin. This will ensure easy removal of the composite after the registration is done.
2. Adjust the composite with a large, pear-shaped, high-speed diamond bur until all posterior teeth are in MIP. Check with articulating paper or film that both the posterior teeth and the anterior stop achieve simultaneous contact on all surfaces (posteriorly on all teeth and anteriorly on the composite stop). Sometimes an equilibration of the posterior teeth is needed (Fig 7-12).

Note: In some cases, multiple-tooth preparation reduces the MMR stability to the point that a condylar support is needed. In such cases, we may need to change our mind about keeping the existing MMR and switch over to creating a new mandibular position (MP) in centric relation (CR) (see chapter 8).

Fig 7-10 Maxillary anterior teeth prepared for full-coverage restorations.

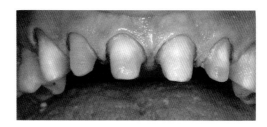

Fig 7-11 Maxillary anterior composite resin stop stabilizing the mandible during the interocclusal registration.

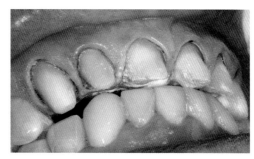

Fig 7-12 Adjust until you have simultaneous stops on the unprepared posterior teeth and on the anterior composite stop(s).

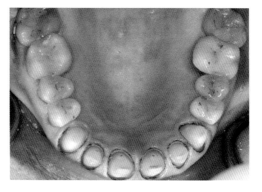

Analog technique

1. Once the teeth are prepared and the desired clearance is achieved, place PVS bite registration paste (Blue Mousse, Futar, etc) or wax in the prepared area, and ask the patient to bite on all teeth (Fig 7-13). Be sure to check that closure is complete, and wait until full setting of the paste or wax before proceeding.
2. Remove the composite resin stop after the interocclusal registration. It is irrelevant to the registration record, since it has a small size relative to the entire record. The occlusal record will fit over the preparation master model, and the "missing" portion of the composite stop, if kept at a minimum, should not impede the fit.
3. Pack and send the impressions and interocclusal registration to the lab.

Digital technique

1. Place the head of the IOS on the right side of the arches, record the interarch relationship, and then repeat the same on the left side. The MMR record is a buccal scan of both arches. The IOS software creates the interocclusal registration in MIP by matching the digital casts of the arches to the buccal scan.
2. Remove the composite resin stop after the interocclusal registration. It is irrelevant to the IOS registration record, since it is "invisible" to the virtual articulated models (Fig 7-14).
3. Upload the digital casts and occlusal record scans to the laboratory's CAD/CAM software.

Fig 7-13 PVS bite registration material applied to the prepared teeth, over the composite stop, to create an analog interocclusal registration.

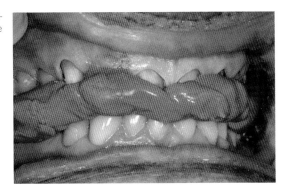

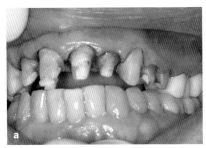 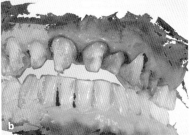

Fig 7-14 *(a and b)* Digital interocclusal registration with an IOS. In the interocclusal registration scan, the composite stop *(in blue)* is "invisible" on the virtual articulated models.

Special Situations

Terminal tooth preparation interocclusal registration

When preparing for a full-coverage crown on the last tooth in the arch, in spite of using occlusal depth cuts and reducing sufficiently, sometimes the reduction seems insufficient—the space has vanished (Fig 7-15). The same can happen when removing an old crown that seemed to have had sufficient reduction. Insufficient reduction may lead to crown fracture during function (Fig 7-16), so we need to be able to identify the cause of this vanishing space.

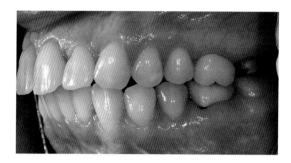

Fig 7-15 The "vanishing space." Sometimes when preparing the last tooth in an arch or removing an old crown, the reduction seems insufficient.

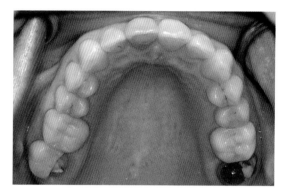

Fig 7-16 This second molar crown cracked within weeks of cementation, and the occlusal reduction appears insufficient.

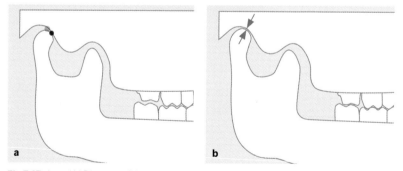

Fig 7-17 *(a and b)* Diagram of the "vanishing space"; the condyle slides up and the occlusal reduction becomes insufficient.

The answer lies with the condyle. When a terminal tooth is prepared, the occlusion between the posteriormost teeth is lost, and the condyle is free to slide upward. Prior to preparation, the CP on the eminence is down and anterior from the fully seated one, and the stability of the mandible is given by the IC. By preparing the occlusal surface of the last tooth in the arch, we allow the condyle to slide up and back, and the space we carefully prepared diminishes as the condyle moves upward (Fig 7-17), giving the impression of a lesser reduction than actually performed.

The best way to prevent this problem is to diagnose the mandibular instability prior to tooth preparation. Limited intercuspal contacts, anterior open bite, and significant wear of the posterior teeth are all risk factors and indications for careful planning of occlusal reduction, even for a single crown. The following steps can be taken to mitigate this risk:

- **Reduce more:** A simple way to ensure sufficient clearance for the restoration is to reduce more of the occlusal surface and/or reduce the opposing dentition.
- **Leave an occlusal stop:** Before preparing the tooth, mark the supporting cusp or surface with articulating paper. Use depth cuts to prepare the entire occlusal surface, leaving the supporting cusp unprepared. Impress or scan the preparation, take the occlusal record (analog or digital), then reduce the unprepared cusp to fit the rest of the occlusal clearance. The technician will make the adjustment of the surface in the lab.
- **Take a pre-preparation scan:** Ask the lab to reproduce the occlusal anatomy and clearance prior to preparation.
- **Equilibrate:** A more elaborate but also more predictable solution is to improve the stability of the mandible. This can be achieved by a complete equilibration, ensuring the simultaneity of the seated CP with the IC. Alternatively, especially in significant anterior open bite situations, a partial equilibration can be performed. Placing the condyles in their fully seated position, the posterior teeth will be adjusted until sufficient occlusal contacts are present. For example, all molars and premolars intercuspate simultaneously with the fully seated CP (see chapter 9).

Implant restoration interocclusal registration

The impression or scan to pick up the position of an implant is different from that of a natural tooth restoration, but the interocclusal registration for the restoration is similar to the single crown technique presented. The main difference is that the impression abutment or the scan body has to be removed because it may interfere with the MIP.

In both the analog and digital workflows, the impression coping or the scan body is removed, and the interocclusal registration is performed with the edentulous space empty (Fig 7-18). When the implant (or implants) is in a terminal position in the arch (Fig 7-19), the situation is similar to the "vanishing space" scenario as well. Because we cannot support the condyle in any way besides bracing it against the eminence, it is recommended to equilibrate the rest of the dentition before the impression or scan. This diminishes the risk of having an implant-supported crown with a prematurity.

Conclusion

Dentists restore in the existing IC in a great majority of clinical situations. By perfecting the techniques presented in this chapter, you will achieve significant time savings. In the analog workflow, remember to trim the recording medium to ensure an accurate articulation of the models. The digital workflow is more accurate in this regard because it uses no recording medium. Also, always use full-arch impressions or scans. Box 7-1 lists some relevant questions and their answers relating to interocclusal registration in the existing occlusion.

Fig 7-18 *(a)* Scan body in place for the implant position scan. *(b)* Scan body removed when capturing the occlusal scan record.

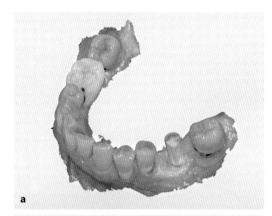

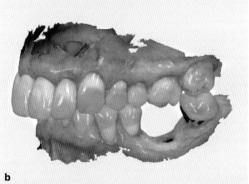

Fig 7-19 Implants in terminal positions in the arch.

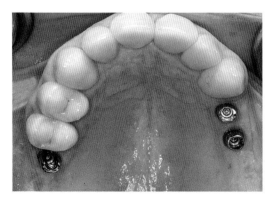

Box 7-1	**Questions and answers about interocclusal registration in existing occlusion**

Q | **Is a "triple tray" easier and quicker because of the single-step process?**

In the analog workflow, it is quicker, but it is also less precise. A digital scan is even quicker and more precise than an analog "triple tray."

Q | **Because most restorations are performed in the existing IC in general practice, can we disregard the MP and record the existing occlusion?**

In a majority of cases, yes. Chapter 8 describes what to do when we have to change the existing occlusion.

Q | **Why is a digital scan occlusal record more precise than an analog one?**

The digital occlusal record has two main advantages: (1) It has no interposed medium potentially changing the MP, and (2) the technician receives the recording precisely reproducing the clinical situation. No manual articulation of the models is required.

Q | **When we can hand-articulate the models, do we still need an occlusal record?**

In the analog workflow, hand articulation of models is many times uncertain; there may be various positions in which the models fit together. When an occlusal record limited to the prepared area is well trimmed, it helps find the best fit of the models, identical to the clinical situation. In the digital workflow, the software can approximate the scans similar to a hand articulation. Instead, the workflow always asks for an occlusal record.

⟶

| Box 7-1 cont. | **Questions and answers about interocclusal registration in existing occlusion** |

Q | **How often do we encounter a "vanishing space"?**

We encounter a "vanishing space" almost every time we have a preparation of a terminal tooth (see section earlier in this chapter). Think about a chair with multiple legs but one shorter leg. The chair will always shift to rest on that short leg, just like the condyle will always slide when stability is lost. Every time there is a slide from the fully seated CP to MIP, this "vanishing space" is a potential outcome. The greater the slide, the greater the chance of the space vanishing.

Q | **Is the digital workflow worth it for cases where we keep the existing IC?**

Yes! The accuracy of digital scans is similar or better than that of analog models, and there are other advantages regarding transmission to the laboratory. However, the main advantage of the digital workflow is the precision of the occlusal record.

References

1. McNeill C (ed). Science and Practice of Occlusion. Chicago: Quintessence, 1997.
2. Wiskott HWA. Fixed Prosthodontics: Principles and Clinics. Chicago: Quintessence, 2011.
3. Beck F, Lettner S, Zupancic Cepic L, Schedle L. Comparison of virtual intersection and occlusal contacts between intraoral and laboratory scans: An in-vivo study. J Clin Med 2023;12:996.

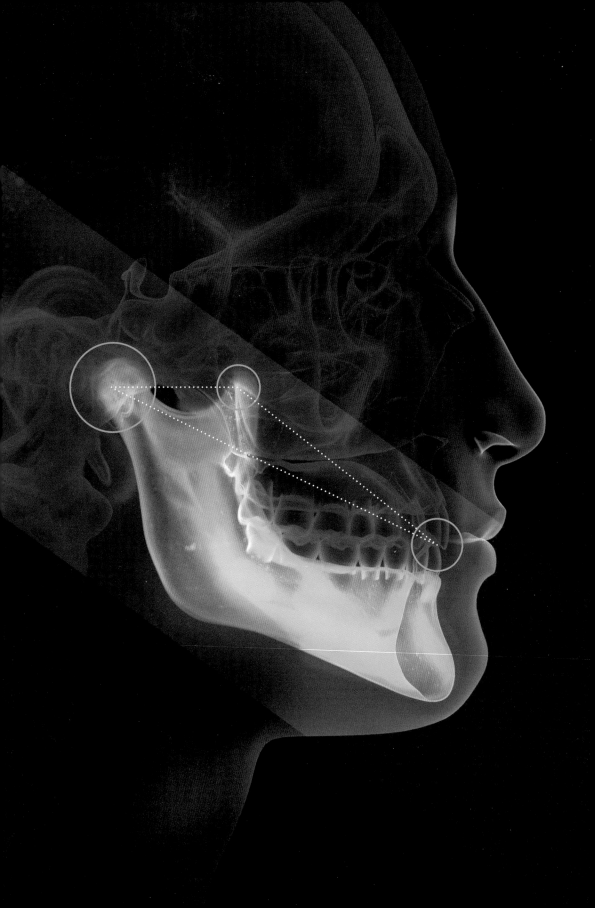

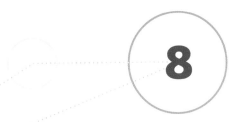

8

Techniques for Interocclusal Registration for a New Occlusion

With contributions from Daniel Radu, DMD

The clinician needs to provide the lab with an interocclusal registration even in cases where there is no existing occlusion or when we decide to change the existing occlusion, such as in the following clinical situations (Fig 8-1):

- Completely edentulous cases with or without implants
- Preparation of all teeth in one or both arches
- Alteration of vertical dimension of occlusion (VDO) for treatment purposes
- Functional changes to the mandibular position (MP)

This is the "problem bite," and the occlusion formula to consider is O = IC + CP + ARP. In all of these scenarios, we have to choose an MP in which to recreate the intercuspation (IC). Then we have to record that MP and send it to the lab to fabricate restorations that will function in that new occlusion—the reorganized occlusion.[1]

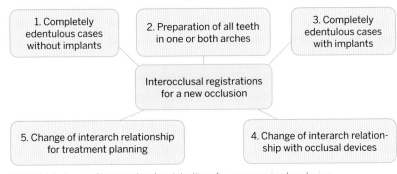

Fig 8-1 Mind map of interocclusal registrations for a reorganized occlusion.

This may seem complicated, because the mandible can assume many positions, but the solution lies in the occlusal formula we discussed in chapter 3. MP is determined by the condylar position (CP) and the anterior reference point (ARP[2]) (see chapter 3):

$$MP = CP + ARP$$
$$O = IC \text{ (given by the lab)} + CP + ARP$$

We can therefore use the CP and ARP to determine a static MP in which to recreate the IC. In certain cases, we may also need to provide the lab a registration of the envelope of function (EoF) for dynamic occlusion (see chapter 10).

This chapter presents a process and workflow for identifying and recording a reorganized occlusion, as well as pitfalls to avoid and particular clinical situations requiring special attention.

General Principles to Apply When Creating a New Occlusion

When creating a reorganized occlusion, the main focus is to find a stable, orthopedically correct MP. We don't record the CP and ARP but the MP given by those landmarks (see Note B).

First, we address the ARP. We create a permissive obstacle[3] (platform or stop) in the anterior area that (1) allows the mandible to travel back and forth and slide side to side, which results in the condyles assuming the orthopedically correct position,[4] and (2) enables the ARP to be adjusted in size and shape to achieve the desired distance to the maxillary incisors or analogs.

Second, we look for the CP. We want to find a CP that is fully seated, physiologic, stable, and reproducible, so it can be a reference position (see Note E). We use physics and biology to do this: When the lateral pterygoid muscles are relaxed, the elevator muscles seat the condyles in their respective fossae (the ball at the bottom of the bowl).

The condyles are the CONSTANT: We do not alter them, only look for their physiologic position. The ARP is the VARIABLE: We construct it as a permissive obstacle, and its shape varies for different clinical situations.

Fig 8-2 Platform on the maxillary arch with all teeth prepared for full-coverage crowns.

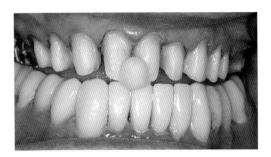

Fig 8-3 To create an accurate registration, avoid full-arch wafers.

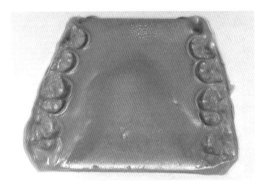

General Workflow for Creating and Recording a New Occlusion

The recommended workflow is as follows (see Note D):

1. Create an anterior obstacle, a sturdy platform on which the mandible can find a definitive stop in closure. This may be done on the maxillary or mandibular arch (Fig 8-2). In an edentulous arch, the platform may be created on an analog (occlusal rim; see Fig 8-8). The result is a tripod between the platform and the condyles (see Fig 3-3), which ensures the stability of the mandible for the recording (one of the principles of recording). The physical registration takes place intraorally, at the level of the arches, using the intraoral tripod. A tripodic interocclusal registration is preferred to one using a full-arch wafer of wax (Fig 8-3).
2. Adjust the platform height to allow for fabrication of the planned restoration or device.

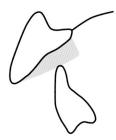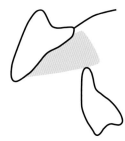

Fig 8-4 Illustration of the mandibular incisal point moving distally when the lateral pterygoid muscle relaxes, creating a large overjet that must be accommodated in the final restoration.

3. Adjust the platform to allow the mandible to travel smoothly back and forth (in the sagittal plane) and side to side (in the horizontal plane) when the patient is directed to perform that movement.

4. Instruct the patient to move the mandible back and forth two to three times and then clench in the posterior position. Because the mandible travels under the action of the elevator and lateral pterygoid muscles, the condyles assume a physiologic, fully seated, stable position in the fossae. This is an individual position created by the specific resultant vector of force of each patient.

5. Check the position of the mandibular central incisors (or analogs) two to three times to observe if the end point of the mandibular movement is repeatably the same.

6. Check the space (clearance) available as a result of closing on the platform. Keep in mind that repeated back-and-forth movement of the mandible relaxes the lateral pterygoid muscles and allows the condyles to travel further posteriorly and superiorly, which may position the incisal point further away from the maxillary teeth (or analogs), thereby increasing the anterior space to be completed by restorations (Fig 8-4). At the same time, the posterior space (clearance) may be diminished, calling for further adjustment there (see Fig 7-17).

This process has two goals: *(1)* find a stable and repeatable MP, and *(2)* ensure that the clearance (anteriorly, posteriorly, and in between) is appropriate for the planned restoration or procedure. When the two goals are met, the MP can be recorded.

Box 8-1	**General workflow for interocclusal registration for a new occlusion**

Anterior
1. Establish/create ARP
2. Adjust to desired VDO
3. Make permissive

Posterior
4. Find CP (centric relation, CR)
5. Verify
6. Record MP
7. Record EoF

Box 8-2	**Clinical situations where a new occlusion must be established**

1. Completely edentulous cases without implants
2. Preparation of all teeth in one or both arches
3. Completely edentulous cases with implants
4. Change of interarch relationship with occlusal devices
5. Change of interarch relationship for treatment planning

7. Record the static MP achieved by the tripod between the anterior platform and the two condyles using an analog or digital workflow. A facebow recording is helpful to the technician (see chapter 11).

The techniques presented in this chapter cover all usual clinical situations with missing IC. The common denominator is the process of finding the stable CP (Box 8-1). The variable is the way we construct the anterior platform and the shape and size of it. While the principle is the same, various clinical situations (Box 8-2) call for various procedures to stabilize the anterior portion of the mandible. As the saying goes, we can be firm in principle and flexible in procedure. The rest of this chapter is dedicated to specific techniques for creating and recording a new occlusion in these clinical situations.

Finding and recording the stable MP is not a quick step. It is a process that needs to be done carefully and methodically, and most of the time it must be repeated until we can validate that we are in the right MP.

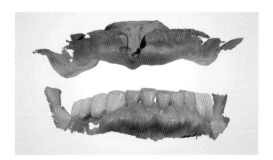

Fig 8-5 Case of edentulous maxilla to be restored with a removable complete denture.

1. Completely Edentulous Cases without Implants

Case example

A 69-year-old woman presented with the desire for a new maxillary denture (Fig 8-5). Her chief complaint was the inability to chew food, even when using denture adhesive. Every time she bit down, the denture had to displace in order to achieve maximal intercuspation (MIP). The treatment plan was to fabricate a new maxillary denture with an emphasis on creating an MIP in harmony with the seated condyles.

Occlusal considerations

Applying the occlusion formula (O = IC + CP + ARP) to an edentulous case, we lack the IC, and the VDO (ie, ARP) and CP are uncertain (Fig 8-6). Because all teeth are missing and the VDO is lost, we have to establish a new IC in a physiologic MP. If possible, we should also communicate the EoF to the lab (see chapter 10).

   The interocclusal registration is critical for treatment success. Many unsuccessful treatment outcomes are related to "missing the bite." Because the denture bases are not attached to the jaws, any force applied to the teeth during function may displace the denture. If the teeth setup is not in harmony with the function, the denture becomes very unstable. We therefore need to change the patient's random MP to a physiologic one (seated condyles at the desired VDO) and recreate the MIP (denture teeth setup) in that relationship. A common pitfall is asking the patient to bite into a softened wax rim, which is prone to inaccuracy (Fig 8-7).

Fig 8-6 Diagram illustrating the missing components of occlusion in the case of an edentulous maxilla.

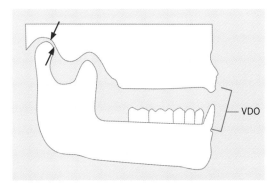

— VDO

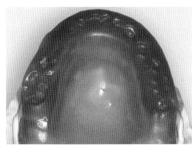

Fig 8-7 The patient's opposing teeth leave indentations in a soft wax rim. This method is prone to inaccuracy when performing interocclusal registration.

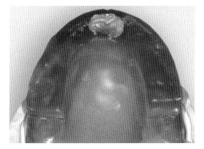

Fig 8-8 Platform on an occlusal rim. This occlusal rim with a hard wax (Delar) creates firm support in the incisor area.

Fig 8-9 The composite platform creates a solid ARP, establishes the desired VDO, and helps find the seated CP.

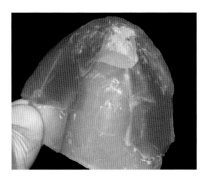

The challenge is to create a defined ARP for the mandible. To ensure a firm and definitive rest of the mandible on the maxillary occlusal rim, we recommend a modified rim with a lingual hard stop (Fig 8-8). This stop is also used to find the stable CP. The hard stop can be a composite platform incorporated into the wax rim (Fig 8-9).

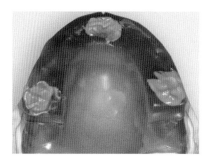

Fig 8-10 Hard wax (Delar) is added to the right and left molar areas and softened. The patient's opposing teeth leave indentations as they close onto the anterior firm stop (platform).

Analog technique

1. Create a maxillary occlusal rim with wax on a base plate of Triad (Dentsply Sirona).
2. Adjust the wax rim to achieve adequate lip support and a horizontal occlusal plane.
3. Adjust the wax rim in the anterior zone to establish the desired VDO; reduce the rim until the mandibular incisors find the desired VDO.
4. Create a firm stop (platform) in the anterior area for the mandibular incisors to rest on. Add a hard wax (Delar; see Fig 8-8) or a composite (Triad) stop (see Fig 8-9). Make sure the other mandibular teeth do not touch the maxillary wax rim; This will ensure a stable tripod between the anterior stop and the condyles.
5. Ask the patient to move the mandible front to back two to three times, while supporting the maxillary occlusal rim with the fingers, and stop in the posterior position. This requires a hard material such as Triad as a stop. Repeat until the patient naturally assumes that position, which can be considered CR. If using only a hard wax (Delar), ask the patient to move the mandible backward and close. Soften the Delar wax and have the patient repeatedly find that position. That will complete the finding of CR at the desired VDO.
6. To record that position, add hard wax (Delar) in the right and left molar areas, and soften it enough so the mandibular teeth can leave an indentation (Fig 8-10).
7. Send the maxillary occlusal rim and the mandibular model or impression to the lab. A facebow record should also be taken and sent to the lab, along with a model of the teeth, preferred shade, and instructions on how to set them up for try-in.

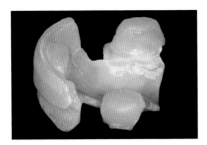

Fig 8-11 Occlusal rim constructed from composite resin (Triad), with cutoffs to allow the scanner to match the image of the edentulous prosthetic field to the opposing arch.

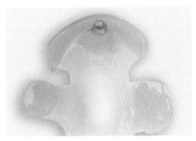

Fig 8-12 Hard wax is added to the anterior zone composite platform for the mandibular incisors to repeatedly access.

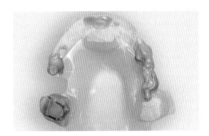

Fig 8-13 Hard wax is added to the posterior areas to stabilize the mandible.

Digital technique

1. Create a maxillary Triad occlusal rim designed with large open cutoffs so the scanner can match the edentulous maxillary arch to the opposing arch (Fig 8-11).
2. Adjust the maxillary rim to achieve adequate lip support and a horizontal occlusal plane.
3. Adjust the Triad rim in the anterior zone to establish the desired VDO; reduce the rim until the mandibular incisors find the desired VDO.
4. Create a firm stop in the area for the mandibular incisors to rest on. Make sure the other mandibular teeth do not touch the maxillary composite rim.
5. Ask the patient to move the mandible front to back two to three times, while supporting the maxillary occlusal rim with the fingers, and stop in the posterior position. Add a hard wax (Delar) on the composite (Triad) stop (Fig 8-12). Repeat until the patient naturally assumes that position, which can be considered CR. Stabilize the mandible by adding Delar wax in the posterior areas as well. This will complete the finding of CR at the desired VDO (Fig 8-13). This finding of the CR

Caution: Note that if you use a full wax occlusal rim, it is hard to achieve a stable MP because the mandible can easily slide once it touches an uneven rim, especially if the contact is in the posterior zone. That is why we suggest the design of the occlusal rim with an anterior contact only; once the stable MP has been established, add the posterior light contacts while checking the anterior stop to ensure the mandible assumes the same position repeatedly.

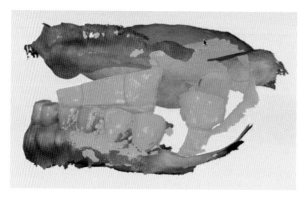

Fig 8-14 Scan of the maxillomandibular relationship.

at the desired VDO is an analog process. The recording that follows is a digital one.

6. Place the scanner to the right and left of the rim and register the interocclusal registration (Fig 8-14).
7. Send all data to the lab.

Variations of the presented case

- *Edentulous mandible opposing a dentate maxilla:* The design of the occlusal rim and process are similar to the one presented.
- *Edentulous maxilla and mandible:* The process is similar to the one presented. The preferred design of the occlusal rims is shown in Fig 8-15. The anterior protuberance is fabricated to substitute for the anterior incisors and used to establish the VDO and find the CR. The posterior protuberances ensure registration of the stable maxillomandibular relationship (Fig 8-16). The relationship between the rims is recorded using polyvinyl siloxane (PVS) paste (Fig 8-17).

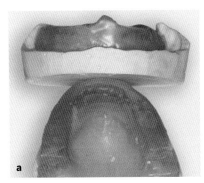
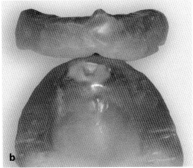

Fig 8-15 *(a and b)* Mandibular occlusal rims modified in the case of edentulism in both arches.

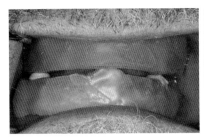
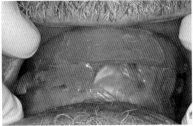

Fig 8-16 Mandibular occlusal rim with three protuberances creating a stable registration.

Fig 8-17 PVS paste is used to record the relationship between the rims.

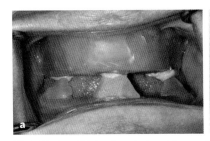
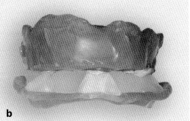

Fig 8-18 *(a and b)* Another design of the maxillary and mandibular rims.

An alternative design of the maxillary and mandibular rims is shown in Fig 8-18. The composite protuberances on the mandibular rim are pointy and create a defined relative position of the two rims without the use of a PVS paste.

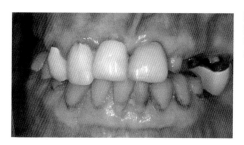

Fig 8-19 Clinical situation requiring extraction of the remaining teeth and fabrication of an immediate complete denture.

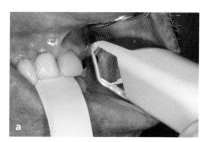 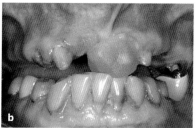

Fig 8-20 *(a and b)* Leaf gauge and composite stop used to establish the desired VDO and find a stable CP.

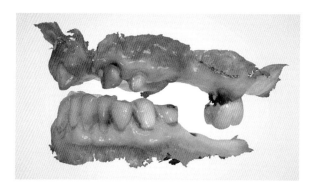

Fig 8-21 Maxillary and mandibular scans digitally "mounted" in CR for the fabrication of a maxillary immediate complete denture.

- *Partially edentulous arches planned for extractions and fabrication of an immediate complete denture*: A typical example is shown in Fig 8-19. Such cases lend themselves to a digital workflow. The interocclusal registration is facilitated by the existence of some teeth that offer a stable reference. If the VDO must be increased, we can use a leaf gauge or a composite stop to stabilize the mandible and facilitate the scan (Fig 8-20). The lab then gets scans mounted in CR at the desired VDO as well as the initial scans to aid design of the immediate denture (Fig 8-21).

Fig 8-22 Diagram of all teeth in one arch requiring restorations. Note the lack of IC, CP, and ARP, meaning we have no components of the occlusion formula.

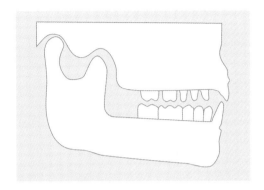

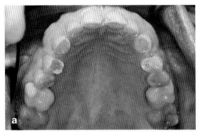

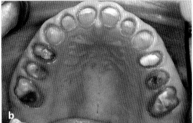

Fig 8-23 *(a)* Maxillary teeth requiring restorations. *(b)* All maxillary teeth are prepared for full coverage. *(c)* The prepared teeth have no definitive relationship with the opposing dentition.

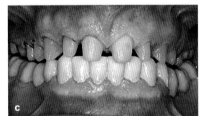

2. Preparation of All Teeth in One or Both Arches

Occlusal considerations

In this clinical scenario, because all teeth are prepared, the existing occlusion or IC is lost, and there is no definitive relationship to the opposing dentition (Fig 8-22). A new MP (ie, CP and ARP) must be established and recorded for the lab. If the patient has healthy muscles and joints, the CP of choice is CR, and the ARP will be at the desired anterior opening. Figure 8-23 shows a representative example of a maxillary arch requiring full preparation and the consequences to the occlusion.

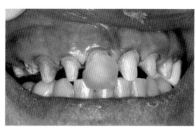

Fig 8-24 Composite resin stop at an approximate VDO on both maxillary central incisors.

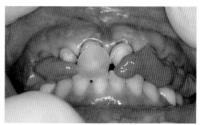

Fig 8-25 PVS paste used in conjunction with the anterior stop to record the maxillo-mandibular relationship.

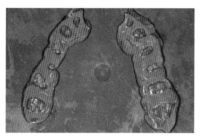

Fig 8-26 Interocclusal PVS wafer trimmed.

Analog technique

1. Fabricate a composite resin stop on one or both maxillary central incisors at an approximate VDO. Make the device out of a light-polymerized composite resin; make it oversized at first and reduce it gradually to the desired height so as to have sufficient occlusal clearance for the design of the fixed prostheses (Fig 8-24).
2. Ask the patient to move the mandible forward and then backward; adjust the device using a diamond rotary instrument (KS4, Brasseler) to allow for smooth movement of the mandible. Repeat this two or three times. When the mandible reaches the backward position, ask the patient to clench and hold that position. This MP is considered CR.
3. A PVS bite registration paste (Blue Mousse, Futar, etc) or wax is placed right and left over the prepared teeth, posterior to the composite stop (Fig 8-25). Wait until complete setting of the paste or wax. The PVS wafers have to be trimmed to the point of leaving only a few clear surfaces for articulation (Fig 8-26).
4. Send the impressions and interocclusal registration to the lab. A facebow record and shade should be taken and sent as well.

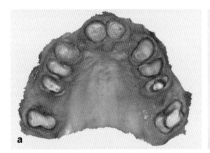 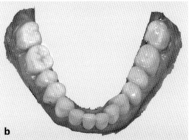

Fig 8-27 *(a and b)* Digital scans of prepared maxillary teeth and mandibular arch.

Fig 8-28 Composite resin stop on the maxillary central incisors. Make it oversized and adjust to the desired anterior opening; also make it "permissive" to allow the mandible to move back and forth, relax the lateral pterygoid muscles, and find CR.

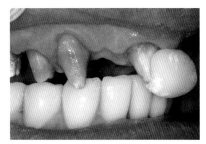

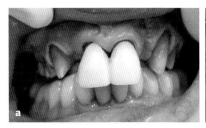 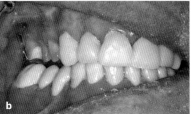

Fig 8-29 A stop at the desired VDO may be an existing provisional restoration. *(a)* Existing provisional restoration of the central incisors. *(b)* Existing provisional restoration of all six anterior teeth.

Digital technique[5]

1. Take scans of the prepared and opposing arch (Fig 8-27).
2. Fabricate a small composite resin stop on one or both maxillary central incisors at an approximate VDO. Make the device out of a light-polymerized composite resin; make it oversized at first and reduce it gradually to the desired height so as to have sufficient occlusal clearance for the design of the fixed prostheses (Fig 8-28). This composite stop may also be an existing provisional restoration (Fig 8-29).

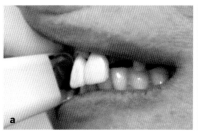 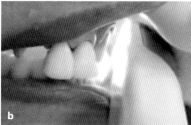

Fig 8-30 *(a and b)* CR recording with the IOS.

3. Ask the patient to move the mandible forward and then backward; adjust the device using a diamond rotary instrument (KS4, Brasseler) to allow for smooth movement of the mandible. Repeat this two or three times. When the mandible reaches the backward position, ask the patient to clench and hold that position. This MP may be considered CR.

4. Place the head of the intraoral scanner (IOS) on the right side of the arches and record the interarch relationship, and then repeat the same on the left side (Fig 8-30). The TRIOS 3 (3Shape) software creates the interocclusal registration, with the mandible placed in CR at the determined VDO (Fig 8-31).

5. Upload the digital casts and occlusal record scans into the CAD/CAM software. The data can then be used to design and fabricate the fixed partial dentures (Fig 8-32).

Note: Find the desired opening at incisor level that ensures sufficient clearance at the molar/premolar level. This will avoid the need to increase the VDO later by changing the pin of the articulator, which could introduce an inaccuracy. When establishing the desired anterior opening, evaluate the clearance of the prepared posterior teeth for potential need of occlusal reduction. The opposing arch may need to be altered as well.

Fig 8-31 *(a and b)* TRIOS 3 software matching digital casts of arches to interarch scan (shown in *light blue*).

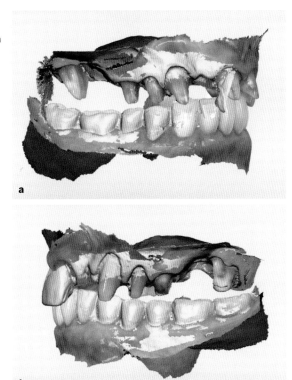

Fig 8-32 Digital CR recording at the desired VDO.

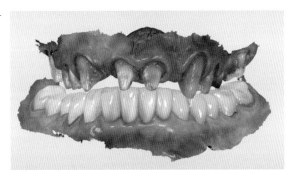

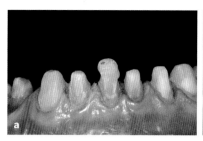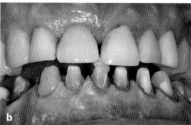

Fig 8-33 *(a and b)* Preparation of the mandibular teeth with the anterior stop on the mandibular central incisor.

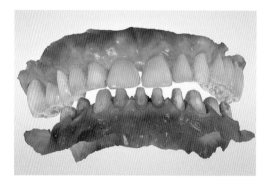

Fig 8-34 Digital CR mounted scans.

Variations of the presented case

- *Preparation of all mandibular teeth opposing a dentate maxilla:* The process is similar to the one described. The anterior composite stop may be fabricated on the prepared mandibular central incisors (Fig 8-33) or on the maxillary central incisors. This helps find and record the CR at the desired anterior opening (Fig 8-34).

- *Preparation of all maxillary and mandibular teeth:* The process is similar to the one described above. The anterior stop (platform) may be fabricated on either the maxillary or mandibular central incisors. If both arches need to be restored, the mandibular arch should be restored first, then the maxillary arch—not the other way around. Ideally, full-arch preparation of both arches should not be done at the same time. The rationale is that the incisal plane of the mandibular arch is a visible landmark and should be established first, and the palatal aspect of the maxillary teeth will fit that plane.

Fig 8-35 Anterior stop placed on the canines because the incisors are missing.

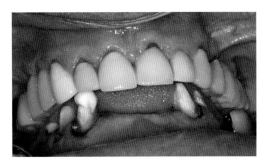

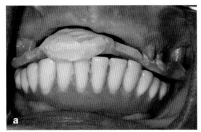
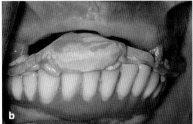

Fig 8-36 *(a)* Anterior stop placed on an occlusal stabilizing wafer (Triad), with Delar wax used for definitive imprints. The premolars are the most anterior teeth present. *(b)* The mandibular teeth are also imprinted in Delar wax.

Other variations are considered a *modified* anterior stop. In other words, the ARP of the mandible may be established in various ways based on the clinical situation. The stable CP is the constant, and the ARP is the variable. The dentist has to be creative and find the optimal technique to stabilize the anterior portion of the mandible.

Modified anterior stops

- *Missing the most anterior teeth (central and/or lateral incisors):* The solution is to place stops on one or both canines—the most anteriorly positioned contact (Fig 8-35). Alternatively, an occlusal stabilizing composite wafer (Triad) can be fabricated and used to record the CR at the desired VDO (Fig 8-36).

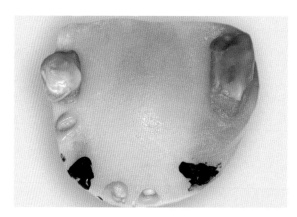

Fig 8-37 Occlusal stabilizing composite wafer (Triad) when multiple teeth are missing. The most anterior aspect of it is used to establish the desired VDO.

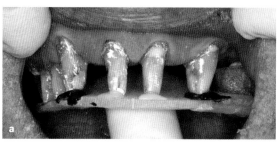

Fig 8-38 *(a and b)* Occlusal stabilizing composite wafer (Triad) adapted to terminal edentulous areas.

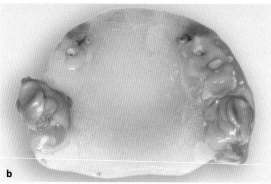

- *Multiple teeth missing and all remaining teeth prepared for restorations:* An occlusal stabilizing composite wafer (Triad) can be fabricated and used to record the CR at the desired VDO (Fig 8-37).
- *Terminal edentulous dentitions with existing prepared anterior teeth:* A similar technique can be done, adapting the Triad plate to the partially edentulous areas (Fig 8-38).

Box 8-3 **Questions and answers about interocclusal registration in a new occlusion**

 Is it helpful to prepare only a few teeth in the arch, record the bite, and then prepare the rest and take another bite?

This process works if we want to keep the existing occlusion, but the technique described in the previous sections is designed specifically for clinical situations where we need to increase the VDO and find a new MP.

 Can we increase the VDO with crowns on the anterior teeth and make composite restorations on the posteriors?

Yes, this is especially helpful when we want to perform a phased treatment. At the time of making the provisional anterior restoration, the posterior teeth can be restored with composite restorations, usually with a single occlusal contact on a holding cusp. When we take the impression or scan for the anterior restoration, we get a complete model and interocclusal registration for the lab. The posterior composite restorations may be replaced with porcelain at a later time, or patients may use the provisionals long-term. However, the composite may wear, and the teeth may supererupt to compensate.

Box 8-3 lists some common questions and answers about interocclusal registration in a new occlusion.

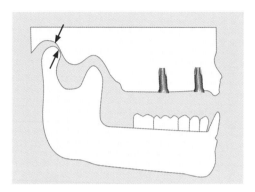

Fig 8-39 Diagram of edentulous arch with implants ready to be restored. Note the lack of IC, CP, and ARP, meaning we have no components of the occlusion formula.

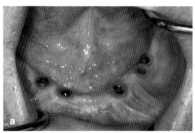 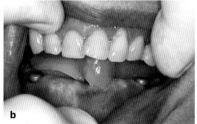

Fig 8-40 *(a)* Typical example of edentulous mandible with implants. *(b)* A firm platform (rest) is created in the incisor area at the most anteriorly placed implant as a permissive obstacle.

3. Completely Edentulous Cases with Implants

Occlusal considerations

In this clinical scenario, because all teeth are missing in one arch, the occlusion or IC is lost, and there is no definitive relationship to the opposing dentition (Fig 8-39). We must create a permissive obstacle to establish the ARP for the mandible using an occlusal rim, composite resin, or other device in the anterior zone (Fig 8-40).

This section presents two clinical situations related to all-on-implants interocclusal registrations—before implant placement and after implants placement. Each one can be done in an analog or a digital workflow. After the implants are placed, it is easier to establish the ARP (VDO), because we now have fixed landmarks (the implants) to stabilize an anterior stop (such as an occlusal rim, composite platform, or other device). There

Fig 8-41 A provisional complete denture is fabricated before the surgery and modified to accommodate the implants.

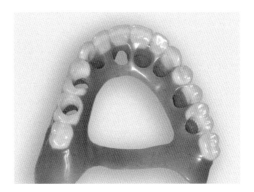

Fig 8-42 After implant placement, the denture is connected to the implants using temporary titanium abutments.

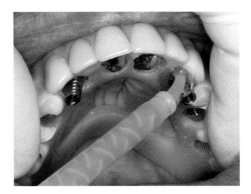

are various approaches and techniques, and more are being developed every day using digital workflows and new materials that allow same-day milling or 3D printing.[6] A few of these techniques are presented here.

Analog technique before implant placement

The steps are identical to the edentulous cases described above; note that in cases where some anterior teeth are present, the planning may be helped by using those as guiding landmarks. A provisional denture is fabricated and will be modified at the time of implant placement (Fig 8-41). This is also called a *reference denture*.[7] At the end of the surgery, temporary titanium abutments are screw retained onto the implants, and the denture is connected to the temporary abutments with composite (Fig 8-42). This process is performed while taking care to maintain the desired position of the mandible.

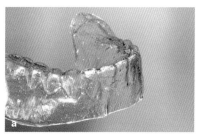
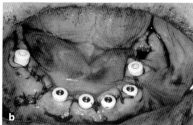
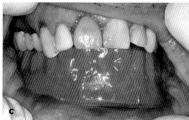

Fig 8-43 *(a)* Vacuum-formed device made over the provisional denture model. *(b)* Healing abutments placed after surgery. *(c)* The vacuum-formed shell is filled with PVS material and placed over the healing abutments and into occlusion with the maxillary teeth.

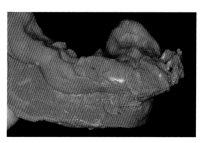

Fig 8-44 An interocclusal registration taken with PVS material between the vacuum-formed shell seated firmly over the healing abutments and the dentition of the opposing arch.

Analog techniques after implant placement

Option 1: Use a vacuum-formed device over the existing or newly made provisional denture

A vacuum-formed device created over the model of the provisional denture is filled with a PVS paste (Futar, Kettenbach) and placed over the healing abutments of the freshly placed implants after suturing the flaps (Fig 8-43). The vacuum-formed shell filled with PVS has to be oriented in the desired vertical, horizontal, and sagittal directions. This may introduce some inaccuracies in the procedure.

After setting of the PVS paste in the shell, another layer of PVS is applied to the occlusal surface, and an interocclusal registration is recorded guiding the mandible in the desired position (Fig 8-44).

Note: This technique can also be used after complete osseointegration of the implants.

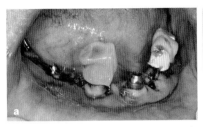
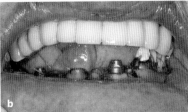

Fig 8-45 *(a and b)* Anterior stop on one anterior implant abutment. The VDO is established using a posterior portion of the provisional restoration.

Fig 8-46 Intaglio surface of the occlusal record displaying the anterior stop picked up in the PVS recording material. The posterior provisional stop was removed prior to applying the PVS paste over the prosthetic field.

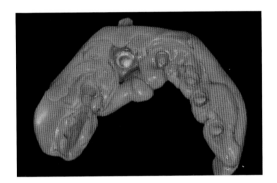

Option 2: Use an occlusal rim with wax on a base plate of Triad

Use the steps from the completely edentulous case. This technique may produce less accurate records due to the potential instability of the support and wax record. This technique is used after osseointegration of the implants.

Option 3: Use an anterior stop created on the most anterior implant

The composite stop has to be adjusted to allow the condyles to be seated, and the height should be at the desired VDO (Fig 8-45). A PVS paste over the anterior stop and the rest of the implant healing abutments will create the interocclusal registration (Fig 8-46).

This method is similar to the preparation of all teeth in one arch, and it may be used immediately after implant placement or after osseointegration.

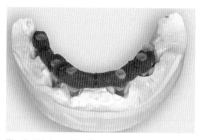

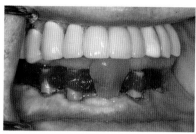

Fig 8-47 A verification jig with plastic abutments connected with pattern resin is made in the lab on the master cast.

Fig 8-48 After ensuring the passive fit of the verification jig, we make a composite (Triad) protrusion to create a platform to establish the VDO and help find the CR.

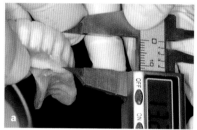

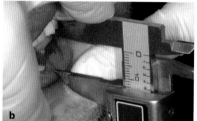

Fig 8-49 (a and b) The VDO of the provisional complete denture is measured and replicated in the height of the anterior jig.

Option 4: Use a verification jig to ensure the accuracy of the impression and precision of the working model

A verification jig can be used to ensure the accuracy of the impression and precision of the working model (Fig 8-47). Add a composite (Triad) protrusion on the jig to establish the desired VDO (Fig 8-48). The same anterior stop will be used to find the CR and stabilize the mandible. To ensure that the VDO of the provisional complete denture is replicated in the anterior jig, we measure it with a micrometer (Fig 8-49). The interocclusal registration is acquired with PVS paste or Delar wax (Fig 8-50). The Delar wax is a rigid wax when cooled and renders a more stable positioning of the working models (Fig 8-51).

Alternatively, when possible, the verification jig can be modified by adding sufficient composite material, adjusted, and used to serve as an interocclusal registration (Fig 8-52). We create a stable tripod between the most anterior point and the two most posterior right and left points.

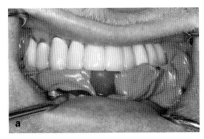
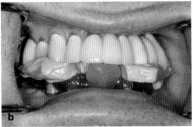

Fig 8-50 An interocclusal registration can be created with PVS paste (*a*) or Delar wax (*b*).

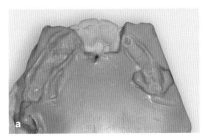
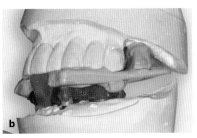

Fig 8-51 (*a and b*) Delar wax interocclusal registration on the maxillary model and mounted between the models.

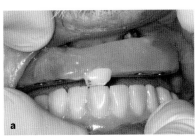
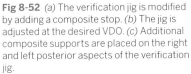

Fig 8-52 (*a*) The verification jig is modified by adding a composite stop. (*b*) The jig is adjusted at the desired VDO. (*c*) Additional composite supports are placed on the right and left posterior aspects of the verification jig.

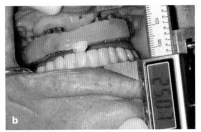
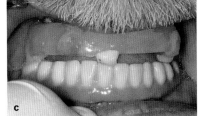

Digital workflow started before implant placement

A CR interocclusal registration is done at the initial appointment, prefer-ably using the present teeth as help to find the stable CP. Again, we do not use the existing IC for this CR record but instead create a stable ARP to find the stable CP using the anterior teeth as support for a composite jig. Planning of the provisional restoration, surgical guide, and final resto-ration will use the initial CR record at the desired anterior opening. This is a hybrid technique using analog impressions but digital interocclusal registrations.

1. Take an analog full-arch pick-up impression using implant impression bodies. After fabrication of the master model, the lab will place scan bodies on the implants and scan with a high-resolution lab scanner to create a digital scan to aid design and fabrication of the restoration.
2. Scan the opposing arch.
3. Measure the existing restorative space with the provisional resto-ration in place (Fig 8-53).
4. On the most anterior implant or implants, insert implant or healing abutments shorter than the desired vertical clearance needed for the restoration. Create a composite stop on those abutments (Fig 8-54), and adjust the composite stop to achieve the desired VDO (Fig 8-55).

The literature is currently divided about the utility of scanning full-arch implants for the purpose of hybrid restorations. Because of the passive fit required by such restorations, existing IOSs are lacking in accuracy. In terms of the interocclusal registrations, however, the accuracy of the scan-ners is adequate.

Fig 8-53 VDO measured with provisional restoration in place.

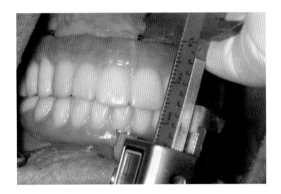

Fig 8-54 An approximate composite (Triad) stop was created over the two most anterior implant abutments.

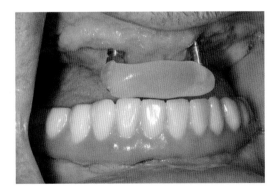

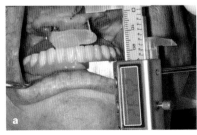
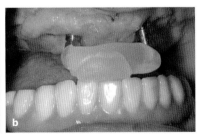

Fig 8-55 *(a)* The VDO is measured with the composite stop, which will be adjusted to reproduce the desired anterior restorative space. *(b)* In this case, composite was added to the initially fabricated stop because the provisional restoration had a larger VDO.

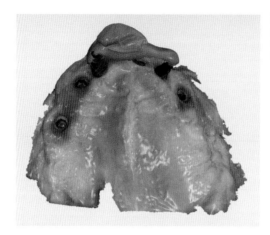

Fig 8-56 An approximate composite (Triad) stop was created over the two most anterior implant abutments.

5. Scan the arch to be restored with the anterior stop in place and with no scan bodies on the posterior implants (Fig 8-56). The precise position of the implants was recorded with the initial PVS or polyether impression using implant impression abutments. Now, we only create the interocclusal registration with a digital workflow.
6. Use an IOS to scan the precisely positioned arches right and left (Fig 8-57).
7. Send all impressions and scans to the lab.

Fig 8-57 *(a)* Use an IOS to record the relative position of the arches both right and left. *(b and c)* Digital interocclusal registration.

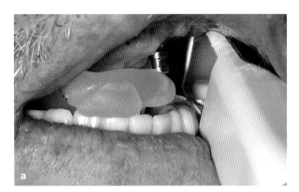

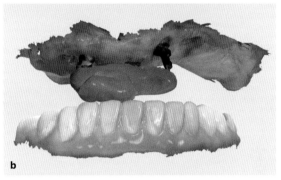

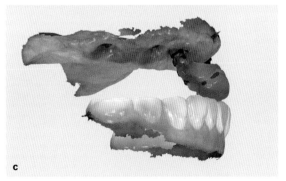

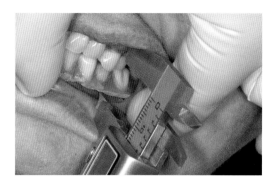

Fig 8-58 The existing VDO is measured with the provisional complete removable denture in place.

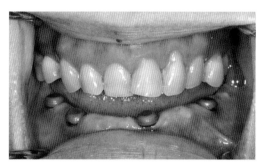

Fig 8-59 Attachments and housings placed over the implants; note the airborne-particle abrasion of the housings to improve scanner accuracy.

Complete digital workflow for restorations with snap-on attachments

Four implants placed in the mandible can be used to stabilize a snap-on complete denture over attachments.

1. A measurement of the desired restorative space is performed using the provisional removable complete denture (Fig 8-58). The attachments and housings are placed over the implants (Fig 8-59).
2. A scan of the prosthetic field is done using an IOS (Fig 8-60), and the opposing arch is also scanned.
3. The housing and attachment on the most anterior implant is removed and replaced with a temporary abutment to create an anterior stop for interocclusal registration (Fig 8-61).
4. A composite (Triad) material is placed over the temporary abutment, shaped as a jig, and cured (Fig 8-62). Using the same technique used for the previously presented cases, the jig is adjusted to the desired VDO and used to find a stable CP (Fig 8-63).

Fig 8-60 Scan of the mandibular arch with the housings placed over the attachments.

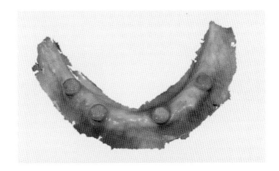

Fig 8-61 A temporary abutment is placed on the most anterior implant.

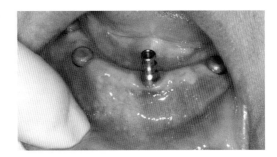

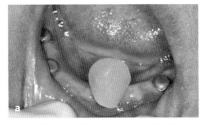 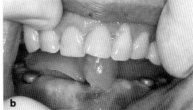

Fig 8-62 *(a and b)* A composite (Triad) stop is placed over the temporary abutment.

Fig 8-63 Composite jig adjusted at the premeasured VDO and used to find the stable CP.

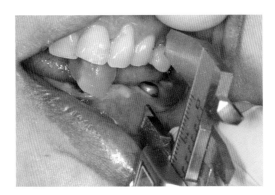

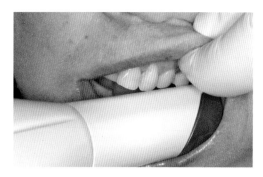

Fig 8-64 Use an IOS to create the interocclusal registration.

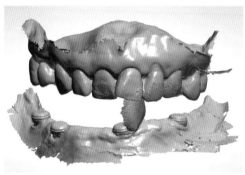

Fig 8-65 Digital interocclusal registration. Note that the anterior composite stop is visible in the occlusion scan but not visible in the virtual mounted scans.

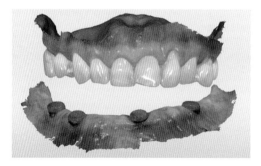

Fig 8-66 Virtually articulated scans used by the lab to fabricate the prosthesis, a mandibular snap-on complete removable denture.

5. After verifying that the mandible repeatedly assumes the same position, ask the patient to hold that position and record it by placing the scanner right and left (Fig 8-64) to create the digital interocclusal registration (Fig 8-65). The virtually articulated scans are used to fabricate the prosthesis (Fig 8-66).
6. All scans are sent to the lab to design and fabricate the restoration.

Important considerations:
- When none of the occlusion factors are present (IC, CP, ARP), finding the desired VDO and CR may be difficult. Multiple rehearsals with the patient and repeated recordings may be needed.
- Avoid recording imprecise (nonrigid) surfaces, such as soft tissue, if possible.
- The accuracy of the interocclusal registrations in edentulous or all-on-implant cases may be less precise than when teeth are present. Be prepared to equilibrate at the time of delivery of the restorations (see chapter 9).

Fig 8-67 Maxillary occlusal device in the mouth.

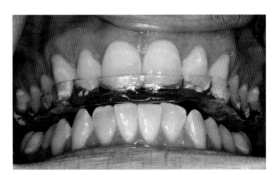

4. Change of Interarch Relationship with Occlusal Devices

Occlusal device is the term used in the Glossary of Prosthodontic Terms for splints, guards, and orthotics (Fig 8-67). Therein, it is defined as "a removable artificial occlusal surface affecting the relationship of the mandible to the maxilla used for diagnosis or therapy."[8] The device may be fabricated on the maxillary or mandibular teeth and is designed to alter the existing IC (see Note G).

This section presents a technique to obtain an interocclusal registration to facilitate the fabrication of an occlusal device in a certain MP. If the clinician desires to fabricate an occlusal device in another MP, the same technique can be used, placing the mandible in the desired position before recording.

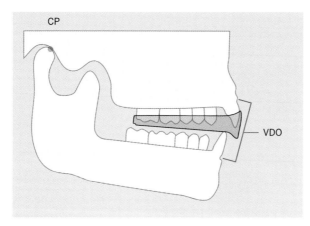

Fig 8-68 Diagram of an occlusal device inserted on the maxillary arch at an increased VDO and allowing the condyles to assume the ortho-pedically stable position in the fossae.

In order to insert a device between the occluding surfaces of the maxillary and mandibular arches, we need to increase the VDO. When we analyze the situation in terms of the occlusal formula (O = IC + CP + ARP), it is clear that we have to decide upon the CP, vertical opening (ARP), and IC. In other words, when we fabricate an occlusal device for a patient, we deal with a "new occlusion" situation (Fig 8-68). This calls for determination of the desired MP similar to the previous techniques in this chapter.

What to avoid: One common way to fabricate the device is to give the impressions or scans of both arches and the MIP interocclusal registration to the lab and ask them to open the articulator arbitrarily to create room for the occlusal device. Another approach is to take a CR record at a random VDO and a facebow recording and then ask the lab to adjust to the desired VDO. Both of these techniques will lead to occlusal devices with imprecise occlusal surfaces that require laborious adjustment chairside.

Fig 8-69 Diagram of a leaf gauge interposed between the incisors as a permissive obstacle.

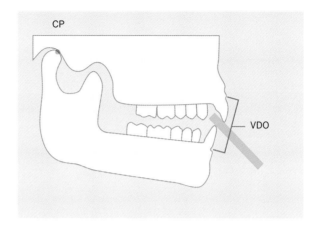

The goals of this process are to obtain the following:

- A recording as close to CR as we can, depending on the state of the masticatory muscles at the time of recording.
- A recording at the desired VDO (ie, sufficient clearance in the posterior area to make a desired minimal thickness of 1 mm). If the lab has to alter the clearance we have recorded, the imprecision of the occlusal fit will be high, even if we have a facebow recording.
- A precise recording so the technician doesn't have to guess or hand-change the interarch relationship.

To accomplish these goals, we recommend a leaf gauge to create a stop/platform in the anterior area of the arches, allowing the condyles to acquire the orthopedically correct position on the eminences (Fig 8-69). If the clinician doesn't have a leaf gauge, an alternative method is to stabilize the mandible by asking the patient to bite on two cotton rolls at the canine level and then record that interarch distance.

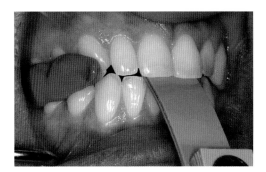

Fig 8-70 CR recording with leaf gauge and PVS paste.

Analog technique

1. Use a leaf gauge and estimate the number of leaves needed to ensure a clearance of no less than 1 mm in the posterior areas. Usually, about 25 leaves or more are needed, depending on the starting relative position of the maxillary and mandibular incisors. If the patient has an anterior open bite, more leaves are needed to disocclude the posterior teeth.
2. Interpose the leaf gauge between the incisors and ask the patient to move the mandible forward and then backward a few times. This will relax the lateral pterygoid muscles.
3. Ask the patient to open wide. Dry the arches with a flow of air, and apply a PVS bite registration paste on the maxillary teeth (right and left separate strands, leaving the front clear).
4. Interpose the leaf gauge and ask the patient to close and move the mandible again back and forth two to three times. When the mandible reaches the backward position, ask the patient to clench and hold that position. This can be considered CR (Fig 8-70).
5. Wait 1 to 2 minutes for the PVS to set, and then remove the two strands of PVS. Trim the material to have only the cusp tips present.
6. Send the impressions and PVS occlusal records to the lab with a prescription for how to design the occlusal device.

Fig 8-71 Leaf gauge used to record CR with an IOS.

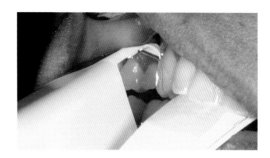

Fig 8-72 TRIOS 3 software matching digital casts of arches to interarch scan (shown in *light blue*).

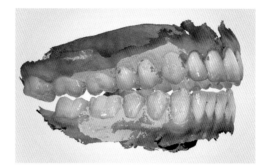

Digital technique[5]

1. Perform steps 1 and 2 of the analog technique.
2. Place the head of the IOS on the right side of the arches and record the interarch relationship, and then repeat the same on the left side (Fig 8-71). The IOS software creates the interocclusal registration with the mandible placed in CR at the determined VDO (Fig 8-72).
3. Upload the digital casts and occlusal record scans into the lab's CAD/CAM software.

Important: The interarch registration for occlusal devices has to relate the MP at an opening that allows the device to be made without opening the articulator any further. Otherwise, because of the difference between patient and articulator, significant occlusal adjustment of the device is necessary at the delivery appointment. Never ask the lab to open the articulator from MIP.

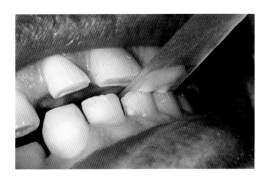

Fig 8-73 Find and record the MP in CR at the projected increased VDO.

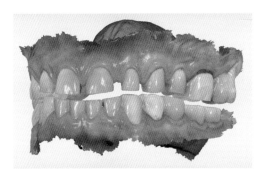

Fig 8-74 Virtual articulation at the desired VDO allows a digital wax-up in the accurate clinical interarch relation.

5. Change of Interarch Relationship for Treatment Planning

When the examination indicates that we must change the occlusion to fulfill the patient's objectives, we need study casts, or scans, mounted in the articulator (see Note F). The future MP must be determined at that time, even if it is just an approximation. If we articulate the casts in MIP and arbitrarily open the articulator, the margin of error is significant. Therefore, the study casts must be articulated in the other reference position available—CR.

We use a similar technique to the one for occlusal devices in CR. The difference is that we estimate what anterior opening we'll need to restore and meet the patient's objectives (Fig 8-73). The wax-up, analog or digital, will be completed in that MP (Fig 8-74), and the provisional restorations will be fabricated from that position, tried in at a mock-up appointment (or at the preparation), and customized. This workflow gets us close to a physiologic MP and reduces the number of adjustments needed.

References

1. Wiskott HWA. Fixed Prosthodontics: Principles and Clinics. Chicago: Quintessence, 2011.
2. Nelson SJ. Wheeler's Dental Anatomy, Physiology and Occlusion, ed 11. St Louis: Elsevier, 2020.
3. Radu, Marandici M, Hottel T. The effect of clenching on condylar position: A vector analysis model. J Prosthet Dent 2004;91:171–179.
4. Okeson JP. Management of Temporomandibular Disorders and Occlusion, ed 8. St Louis: Elsevier, 2019.
5. Radu M, Radu D, Abboud M. Digital recording of a conventionally determined centric relation: A technique using an intraoral scanner. J Prosthet Dent 2020;123:228–231.
6. Antonopoulou S, Cho SH, Kesterke M, Kontogiorgos E, Korentzelos D. Effect of different storage conditions on the fit of 3D-printed occlusal devices used to treat temporomandibular disorders. J Prosthet Dent 2022;128:488.e1–488.e9.
7. Scherer M. The "Reference Denture Technique." https://learndentistry.com/reference-denture-technique/. Accessed 30 December 2022.
8. The Glossary of Prosthodontic Terms: Ninth Edition. J Prosthet Dent 2017; 117(5S):e1–e105.

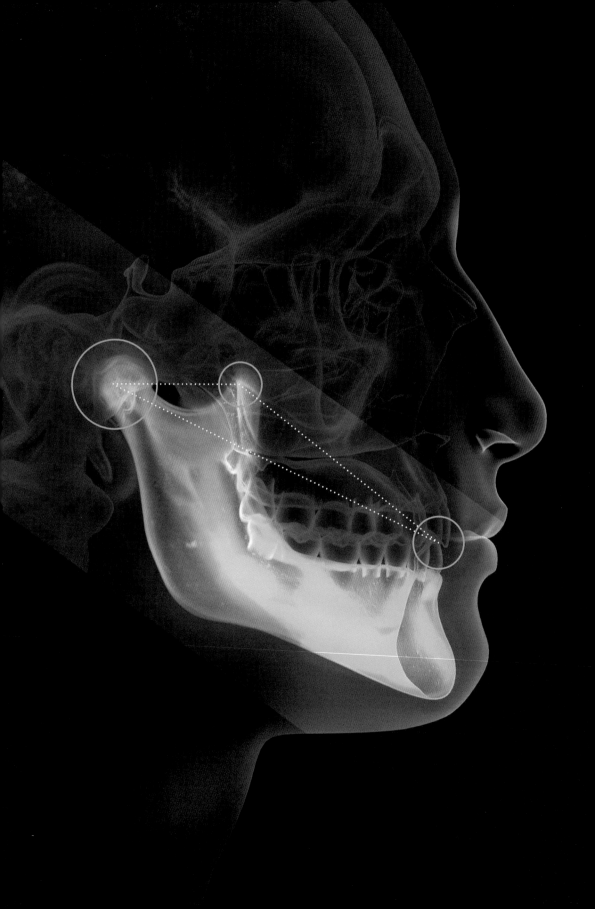

9

Techniques for Equilibration of the Occlusion

"Adjusting the bite" is often a main concern for dentists when performing direct or indirect restorations. Many times, the primary criterion is how it feels for the patient. We keep checking with articulating paper and making adjustments until we feel confident the patient can get used to the new restoration. But that's not always the case, and we need to be careful not to rely on the adaptability of the stomatognathic system to overcome an instability (see Note D).

Why Equilibration Matters

When it comes to occlusion, the difference between very good and very bad is very small—a slight contact can put the entire system out of function. Equilibration is the bridge between that very bad and very good. The goals of equilibration are threefold: *(1)* to create a stable occlusion, *(2)* to minimize forces applied to teeth, and *(3)* to reduce need for adaptation.[1,2]

Consider this case example. A 45-year-old woman presented to my office after more than 2 years of muscle and joint pain following treatment with a beautiful full-mouth restoration at a different dental practice. Over the course of those 2 years, the treating dentist provided an occlusal device and equilibrated the newly delivered restoration many times, with no success. The patient was experiencing nearly constant headaches, muscle and joint pain, and constant preoccupation with her teeth to the point that it was suggested she see a psychologist. Instead she came to our practice looking for help.

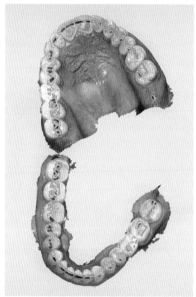 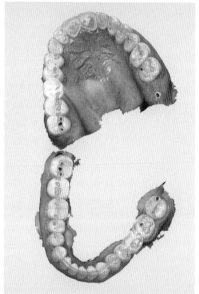

Fig 9-1 Analysis on scans. The maximal intercuspation in habitual occlusion seems perfect.

Fig 9-2 The CR registration using a leaf gauge found a prematurity on the maxillary right second molar on an inclined plane.

Her examination revealed some tender muscles and slight tension of the right joint upon loading. The digital occlusal analysis done with scans and interocclusal registrations showed an almost ideal intercuspation (IC) in her habitual occlusion (Fig 9-1). The centric relation (CR) registration showed a prematurity on the right second molar, with a slide of 1 mm to the right and forward (Fig 9-2). The patient had an occlusal device adjusted by the dentist who did the restoration, but the analysis showed it was not adjusted enough to provide coincidence of CR with maximal intercuspation (MIP) on the device. The patient reported that no bimanual manipulation or leaf gauge was used in the process of adjusting the device.

We adjusted the occlusion with a leaf gauge, and in three appointments over 3 weeks the symptoms subsided completely. At that time we proceeded with an equilibration of the restorations using an anterior composite jig (Fig 9-3). The digital scans showed improvement of the IC in CR (Fig 9-4). We equilibrated once more 1 week later (Fig 9-5), and

Fig 9-3 Anterior composite jig used to equilibrate the restoration.

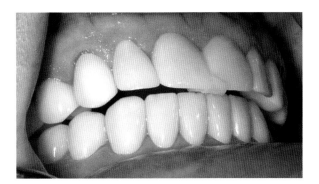

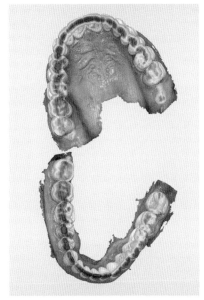

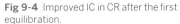

Fig 9-4 Improved IC in CR after the first equilibration.

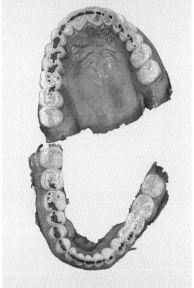

Fig 9-5 The IC after the second equilibration visit.

the patient reported that all symptoms resolved and she felt "perfect." We noticed that the IC was not ideal, but there was no prematurity on the molars. She was scheduled for another appointment but canceled it because she felt no need for it.

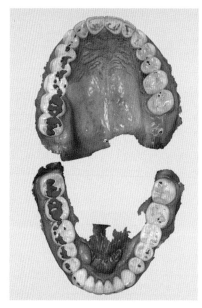 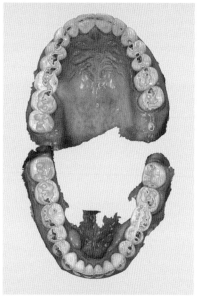

Fig 9-6 The IC 11 months later; note the heavier contacts on the right.

Fig 9-7 IC after reducing the heavy contacts.

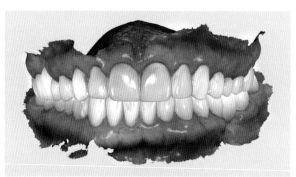

Fig 9-8 Frontal view of IC at 11 months.

Eleven months later she was checked again. She reported that she had no symptoms but that the bite felt heavier on the right side. The scan showed that she was correct (Fig 9-6), so we reduced the surfaces of contact, and 3 months later she once again reported that everything was perfect (Figs 9-7 and 9-8).

The Two Types of Equilibration

The occlusion formula—occlusion (O) = intercuspation (IC) + mandibular position (MP)—has a direct clinical correlation and clarifies the occlusal adjustment or equilibration. We can change only the IC or both the IC and MP, and the adjustment is different for each:

- We can keep the existing occlusion and modify only the new restoration (direct or indirect, single or multiple teeth) to fit with the rest of the teeth. This is considered limited occlusal adjustment, or reshaping.
- We can create a new IC in a new MP by modifying the natural teeth or the restorations. The new MP is given by a stable condylar position (CP), such as CR. The new IC will be achieved by reshaping the existing teeth and/or restorations by ablation. This is considered complete occlusal adjustment, or equilibration.

Therefore, there are two types of equilibration, one limited to the newly inserted restoration and one in which we adjust the natural dentition and/or newly inserted restorations to fit a stable CP. When we keep the existing IC, we harmonize the restoration with the rest of the dentition. When we create a new bite, we harmonize the restoration both with the seated CP and the opposing dentition.

There is a third option: Selective grinding of the opposing dentition without changing the existing occlusion (conformative bite) is indicated in some clinical situations. This creates a better occlusal plane and prevents excursive prematurities.

Limited occlusal adjustment (reshaping)

Reshaping a new restoration is a fairly straightforward procedure that dentists perform daily. Still, some guidelines are worth mentioning.

What you should do:
- Test the closure movement first. This will simplify the process and shorten the time required for reshaping.
- Make sure the mark or marks are on a cusp tip or on a ridge. When the contacts in closure are on inclined planes, the tooth is subject to a lateral force and may drift. Adjust until you achieve this goal (Fig 9-9).
- Test the excursive movements (laterotrusion and protrusion). If needed, adjust the new restoration until it is in harmony with the rest of the dentition. In other words, the new restoration should have similar marks as the adjacent teeth in excursive movements of the mandible.
- Special care should be taken for implant-supported crowns (fixed partial dentures). Due to lack of intrusion of the implants, the restorations should be about 50 microns in infraocclusion.
- Use fine diamond burs and polish adjusted surfaces to high gloss.

What you should avoid:
- When adjusting the most posterior tooth in the arch, make sure the occlusal stop is not on the mesial aspect of a cusp, because that will cause distalization of the tooth and result in an open interproximal contact (Fig 9-10). A contact on the distal aspect of a cusp will help prevent an open contact.

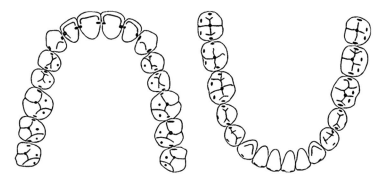

Fig 9-9 Ideal occlusal contacts.

Fig 9-10 *(a and b)* Contact on the mesial aspect will cause the most posterior tooth in an arch to migrate distally and open the contact point.

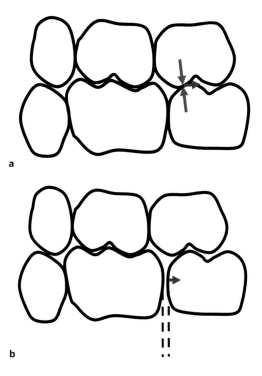

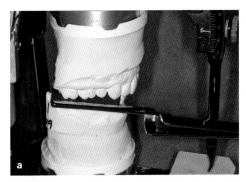

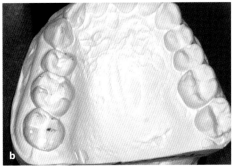

Fig 9-11 *(a)* Equilibration on models mounted in CR. *(b)* Prematurity (first contact) mark on the second molar.

Complete occlusal adjustment (equilibration)

Complete equilibration may be indicated in the following clinical situations: when occlusal devices are used (because they inherently change the MP), to harmonize the natural dentition with the seated CP, and when full-arch restorations (fixed or removable partial dentures with or without implants) are used. Although studies show that an equilibrated occlusion may revert to acquiring a slide from CR to MIP,[3] we should always strive to create a stable system at the end of extensive restorative procedures. Even if the joints and teeth adapt over time, it is helpful to give the stomatognathic system a state of stability at the end of extensive treatment rather than hope the adaptability will reestablish the stability.[4]

It is advisable and prudent to practice full-arch equilibration on mounted models first—a trial equilibration (Fig 9-11)—to help envision the process from start to finish. Another way to practice is to equilibrate occlusal devices. The principles are the same as for natural teeth.

It is critical to emphasize that we do not advocate creating an IC simultaneous with the fully seated CP in all cases. Nonetheless, some clinical situations may warrant this goal: patients with full-arch restorations, patients who had their symptoms subside with occlusal device therapy and suffer relapse when not wearing the device, and large orthodontic cases at the end of treatment.

The steps of complete equilibration

1. Test the closure movement

Equilibration begins by testing the closure movement. To do so, interpose an anterior obstacle, such as a leaf gauge, in between the incisors to create a complete disocclusion of all posterior teeth distal to the obstacle. This ensures the creation of a tripod between the two condyles and the anterior obstacle.

The number of leaves needed to create the stable tripod varies greatly, depending upon the clinical situation. In some cases, as few as four to six leaves is enough; other times, when the existing IC occurs with the condyles down the eminence, as many as 20 to 30 leaves are needed to create the posterior disocclusion. (For reference, 10 leaves is about 0.8 mm thick.) Those situations in cases of natural dentition may not lend themselves to equilibration, and other treatment modalities such as orthodontics or restorative work may be needed.

Ask the patient to move the mandible back and forth three to four times on the leaf gauge. This relaxes the lateral pterygoid muscles and prevents the patient from holding the condyles down the eminences. Then ask the patient to clench on the anterior obstacle after reaching the back position during the back-and-forth movement. This ensures that the elevator muscles will seat the condyles in an orthopedically correct, stable position on the eminences. Make sure the posterior teeth are out of contact before proceeding to the next step (use shim stock foil or articulating paper or film).

Reduce the height of the anterior obstacle progressively and check the posterior teeth for contact with the articulating film. Adjust the posterior teeth repeatedly, while reducing the anterior obstacle, until all teeth intercuspate simultaneously with the seated CP. This may take multiple adjustments and may require repeated checking with the articulating film. Adjust each contact to ensure that occlusal stops are on cusp tips or flat surfaces (not on cusp inclines). Repeat the process until all teeth have occlusal stops in desired areas, with one leaf still between the front teeth to allow for freedom of movement.

2. Test the excursive movements

Next, the excursive movements must be tested. To accomplish this, ask the patient to move their mandible forward and sideways (without a leaf gauge interposed or occlusal device) to customize the excursive marks on the anterior and posterior crowns (dynamic occlusion). You want posterior disocclusion by anterior and canine guidance and anterior guidance in harmony with the envelope of function (EoF). This will create dots on the posterior teeth and lines on the anterior teeth (Fig 9-12).

Fig 9-12 *(a)* Dots on the posterior crowns and lines on the anterior crowns from excursive movements of new restorations. *(b)* Dots in the back and lines in the front after equilibration on an occlusal device.

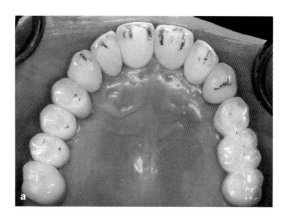

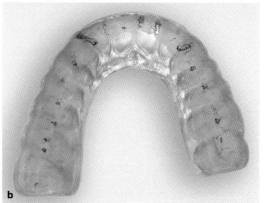

Note: The patient should assume a reclined position in the dental chair during occlusal adjustments because it helps the condyles acquire the fully seated position. At the end of the process, we sit the patient upright and adjust the anterior teeth to ensure even contacts are given in that position. This is called adjusting for "long centric."[5]

Box 9-1	**Guidelines and recommendations for complete equilibration**

- Do NOT attempt occlusal adjustment in full-arch cases without a leaf gauge or another way to create a seated CP to ensure the stability of the mandible. The patient will close randomly due to loss of the previous MIP, which will lead to incorrect adjustments followed by mandibular instability, potential temporomandibular joint problems, and an unhappy patient.
- All fully edentulous cases (with or without implants) are similar to a full arch of crown restorations, and the same rules apply.
- When using a leaf gauge in the case of a complete denture, hold the denture firmly on the prosthetic field.
- Occlusal device adjustments are very similar to those for the natural dentition. An occlusal device has the goal of establishing harmonious occlusal contacts on the device while the patient is wearing it. Because of that, the same rules for IC (in closure and excursions) in the natural dentition apply.
- Always use a leaf gauge or another way to create a seated CP when adjusting an occlusal device.
- When adjusting natural dentition, be mindful of the irreversibility of removal of tooth structure.
- When adjusting occlusion on newly fabricated full-arch restorations, the crowns (fixed partial dentures) must be customized at the time of cementation. Even if the EoF was customized on the provisional restorations, recorded for the lab, and used as the basis for the restorations, because of the many variables involved, the occlusion must be customized intraorally. First make sure the lab has properly designed the occlusal contacts in harmony with the stable MP before cementation and adjust if needed. Then perform the final adjustment after cementation of the crowns because the restorations are now stable on the prepared teeth.

Box 9-1 lists important guidelines and recommendations for complete equilibration.

Fig 9-13 *(a and b)*
Digital equilibration.
Maxillary and mandib-
ular scans articulated
in CR and with a digital
articulator lowered
pin to achieve anterior
coupling.

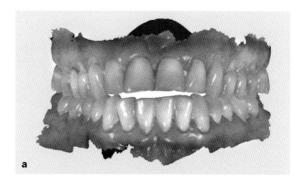

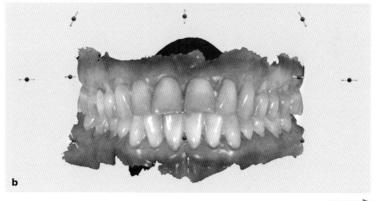

Digital Trial Equilibration

The evaluation of an equilibration on mounted models can be performed on scans digitally mounted in CR on a virtual articulator.

The analog trial equilibration involves pouring the impressions, trimming the models, mounting with a facebow, and performing the equilibration on the stone casts. This may take 1 to 2 hours and must be performed after the patient has left the office.

The digital workflow involves scanning both arches, taking a CR interocclusal registration, and mounting it in a virtual articulator. The articulator pin is dropped until the anterior teeth are in contact, and the "intersections" of the scans in the posterior zone are evaluated (Fig 9-13). The

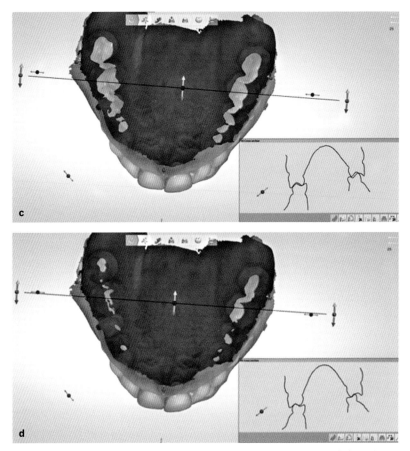

Fig 9-13 *(cont) (c)* Digital articulation showing the amount of reduction needed to achieve anterior coupling ("intersection" of models). *(d)* Less reduction achieves incomplete anterior coupling.

amount of reduction needed is visualized, and the reduction itself can be performed virtually to analyze the resulting occlusal anatomy. The digital process can be done while the patient is still in the chair and takes about 10 minutes.

With the help of the digitally mounted scans, we can visualize and mark the amount needed to be adjusted on each cusp incline, giving us a map of where and how much reduction we have to perform. A template can also be digitally designed, printed, and used to perform the reduction precisely (Fig 9-14).

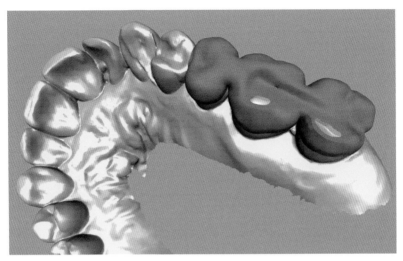

Fig 9-14 A digitally designed template to be printed and used intraorally for precise and quick equilibration.

References

1. Schuyler CH. Equilibration of natural dentition. J Prosthet Dent 1973;30(4 pt 2): 506–509.
2. McCoy G. Dental compression syndrome: A new look at an old disease. J Oral Implantol 1999;25:35–49.
3. Celenza FV. The centric position: Replacement and character. J Prosthet Dent 1973;30(4 pt 2):591–598.
4. Thimmappa M, Katarya V, Parekh I. Philosophies of full mouth rehabilitation: A systematic review of clinical studies. J Indian Prosthodont Soc 2021;21:19–27.
5. Dawson PE. Functional Occlusion: From TMJ to Smile Design. St Louis: Mosby Elsevier, 2007.

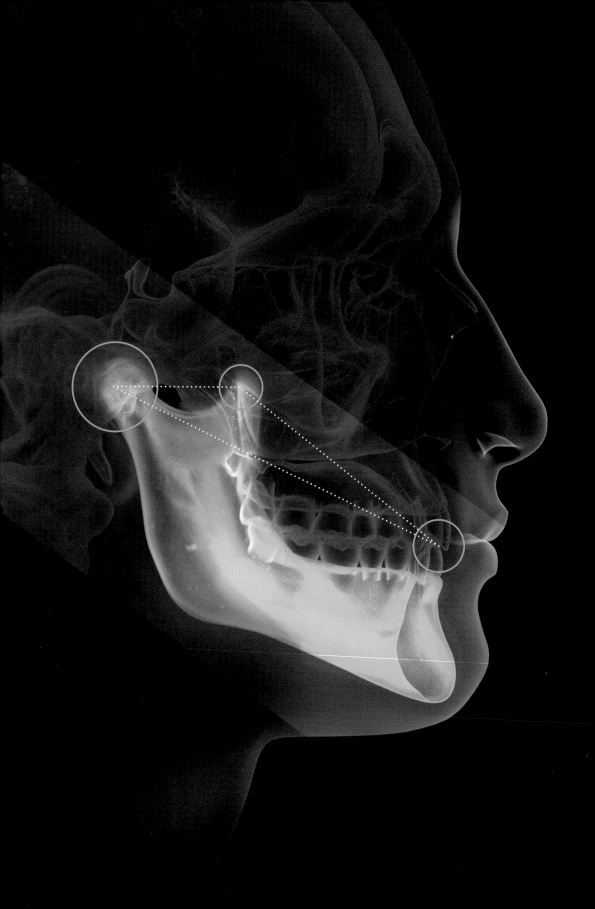

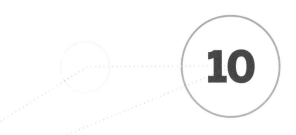

Techniques for Recording the Envelope of Function

The previous technique chapters have presented recordings of static occlusion—that is, the way the mandibular teeth close onto the maxillary teeth at a defined mandibular position (MP). A dynamic occlusion, on the other hand, relates to a mandible in motion, either in function or parafunction, and refers to the way the teeth contact one another during mandibular movement. Recording dynamic occlusion for the lab will facilitate more accurate design and manufacture of restorations and significantly reduce or even eliminate the need for intraoral adjustments.

For practical purposes of communication between the clinician and the lab, the dynamic occlusion may be equated to the envelope of function (EoF), defined as the 3D space within the envelope of motion that determines mandibular movement during function.[1] A simple rule of dynamic occlusion is that only the anterior teeth (incisors and canines) should have contacts in excursions (Fig 10-1). To be more precise, the shape of the palatal aspect of the maxillary anterior teeth (anterior guidance) should be in harmony with the EoF and disocclude the posterior teeth. The contact of teeth during mandibular movement (the dynamic occlusion) will provide the anatomical shape that the lab will copy and reproduce in the final restorations. As such, it is vital that the provisional restorations are tested for function and adjusted as necessary (Fig 10-2).

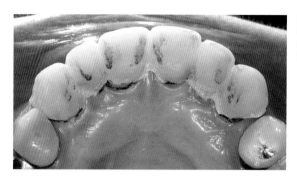

Fig 10-1 Provisional crowns customized on maxillary anterior teeth (anterior guidance).

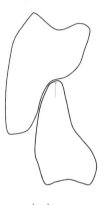 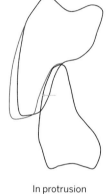

Fig 10-2 Maxillary provisional reshaped and adjusted *(in red)* to allow for mandibular protrusion. As we thin the palatal aspect, we need to add to the buccal aspect to maintain the structural integrity of the restoration.

In closure   In protrusion

The EoF can only be established by the patient's mandibular movements. Even the best articulator cannot reproduce the functional movements of the mandible and the anatomical shapes those movements produce on the opposing teeth. The arbitrary values of the articulator are unable to reproduce the individual pathways of the mandible; those are determined by the masticatory and perioral muscles, ligaments, articular surfaces, and habits of the patient.

This chapter describes how to record the EoF in several patient scenarios, because the last thing you want is a set of restorations that are beautiful and fit perfectly but do not function within the patient's stomatognathic system.

Recording EoF in Cases of Existing Occlusion

When we choose to create a restoration in the existing occlusion, information regarding the dynamic occlusion may appear superfluous. After all, the technician can just use the adjacent teeth and mimic the articulating surfaces, right? Wrong. In reality, even in a single-tooth restoration, the excursive movements of the mandible may be unpredictable, leading to multiple adjustments in the mouth.

Single-tooth preparation

Analog workflow

The clinician should always take a full-arch impression; that will give the laboratory an opportunity to mimic the anatomy of the existing teeth and predict the pathways of mandibular motion.

Digital workflow

When the anatomy is still present, the clinician may take a preparation scan for the lab to predictably create the occlusal (articulating) surfaces. Some oral scanners (eg, TRIOS) even allow the clinician to record patient-specific motion, which can then be sent to the lab along with the preparation and occlusion scan.

Preparation of multiple teeth

See details in "Recording EoF for Preparation of All Teeth in One or Both Arches" on the next page.

Recording EoF in Edentulous Cases with Complete Dentures

When treating an edentulous patient with a complete denture, the EoF is elusive. If the patient has an acceptable old denture, we may record the EoF by copying the occlusal shape of it. Superimpositions over scans are not useful in this patient scenario because the vertical dimension of occlusion (VDO) and MP are most likely far from ideal.

A possible way to customize the EoF is to remount the case after completion and use an articulator to imitate the mandibular movements.

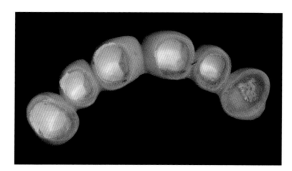

Fig 10-3 Upon removal of these provisional restorations, the temporary cement shows signs of washout on the canine crowns, indicating that the canine guidance should be checked and probably adjusted.

Recording EoF for Preparation of All Teeth in One or Both Arches

Taking the time to perfect the EoF during provisional restoration fabrication saves a lot of time at delivery and avoids the need for costly adjustments, resurfacing, or remakes. The provisional will serve as a template for the final restoration, so it's always best to get the provisional right.

As mentioned earlier, no articulator settings can reproduce and no technician can guess the patient's mandibular movements. Because of that, the clinician must customize the provisionals and make adjustments as necessary until the patient is satisfied and can function well. A good indication that the EoF is precisely customized is the integrity of the provisionals after 3 to 7 days, combined with the retention of the temporary cement; ie, the provisionals do not come loose, and upon removal the cement layer on the intaglio surface is even (Fig 10-3).

The analog workflow

A wax-up is prepared on models mounted in centric relation (CR), improving upon the esthetics if needed (Fig 10-4). The model is then duplicated to allow fabrication of a putty matrix. The provisionals are fabricated in the patient's mouth or on a model (Fig 10-5), fitted over the prepared teeth,

Fig 10-4 A wax-up restores the anatomy and function of the maxillary teeth in CR.

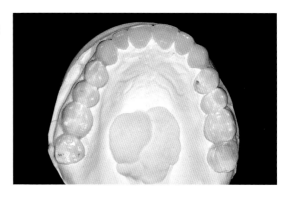

Fig 10-5 Provisionals fabricated intraorally.

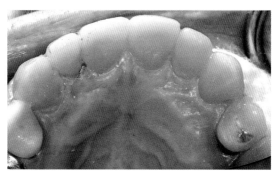

Fig 10-6 The anterior guidance is adjusted in harmony with the EoF.

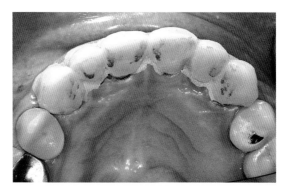

and adjusted in CR using a leaf gauge or bimanual manipulation. The anterior guidance must be established precisely in order to reproduce it in the final restoration (Fig 10-6). In the case of a full-arch preparation, all excursive movements are adjusted to achieve simultaneous centric stops

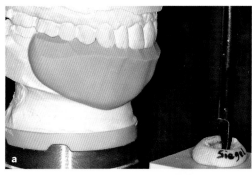

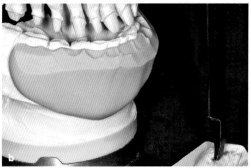

Fig 10-7 *(a and b)* Putty index for the incisal edge position and custom anterior guide table for copying the anatomy of the palatal surface of the maxillary crowns.

and disocclusion through the anterior guidance (dots in the back, lines in the front). A study model of the provisionals mounted in the articulator is then used to create putty indexes (Fig 10-7a). A custom anterior guide table provides the anterior guidance information to the lab[2,3] (Fig 10-7b).

The digital workflow

A digital wax-up is prepared on scans mounted in CR (Fig 10-8). Provisionals can be fabricated using either a printed model (like in the analog workflow) or 3D printing. With 3D printing, shells can be created for relining (Fig 10-9), or the preparations can be scanned and provisionals printed with a fitting intaglio surface (Fig 10-10).

The provisionals must be adjusted or customized to fit the EoF. The same care must be taken as in the analog workflow, sometimes requiring multiple appointments to ensure the customization. However, in the digital workflow this customization takes less time because the provisionals are easier to fabricate.

Fig 10-8 Digital wax-up.

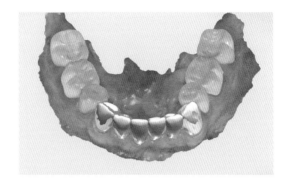

Fig 10-9 Provisional shells printed. These will require fitting on the preparations, relining, and occlusal adjustments.

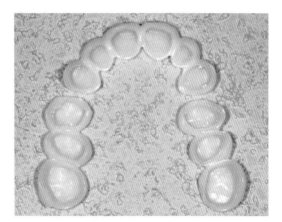

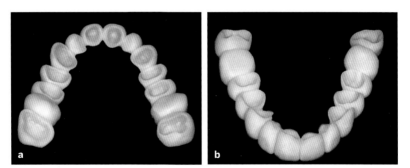

Fig 10-10 *(a and b)* Provisional printed after scanning the preparation of the maxillary teeth. Minimal adjustments will be needed.

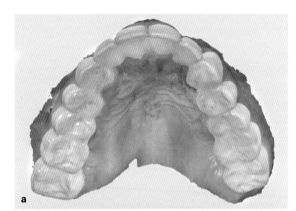

Fig 10-11 *(a)* Scan of customized provisionals. *(b)* Merging of the preparation and provisional scans.

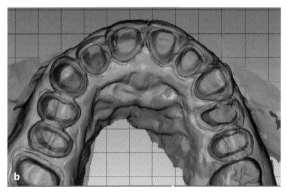

The greatest advantage of the digital workflow is the ease of copying and relating the customized provisionals to the laboratory. A scan of the provisionals can be sent to the lab and merged with the preparation scan (Fig 10-11). For better merging of the scans, segmental scans of the provisionals and preparations may be performed, which facilitates more predictable merging because it relies on hard tissues rather than soft tissue gingiva matching (Figs 10-12 and 10-13).

Jaw-tracking devices: A number of electronic devices have been developed for the purpose of recording the mandibular movement and incorporating it into the virtual articulator. While these devices can be useful, they are difficult to use, time-consuming, and expensive. When we change the occlusion (eg, by increasing the vertical dimension of occlusion [VDO]), we need to test it with customized provisional restorations. These electronic devices can be used in conjunction with the customized provisionals to record the mandibular movements on those provisionals. Furthermore, when we change the occlusion, the old EoF is no longer useful, and we need to establish the EoF in the new MP.

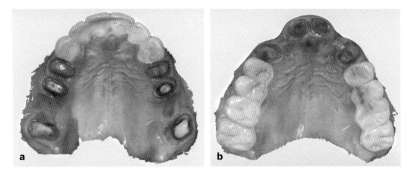

Fig 10-12 *(a and b)* Segmental scans are taken to allow matching of hard structures (teeth and provisionals).

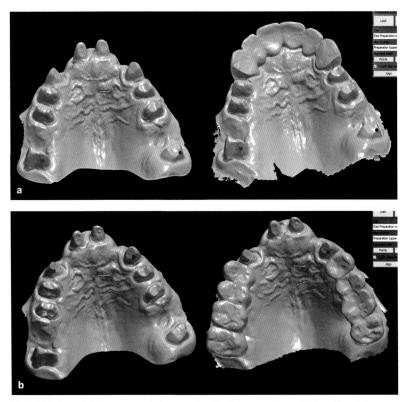

Fig 10-13 *(a and b)* The segmental scans allow the lab a precise matching of hard structures rather than using soft tissue points.

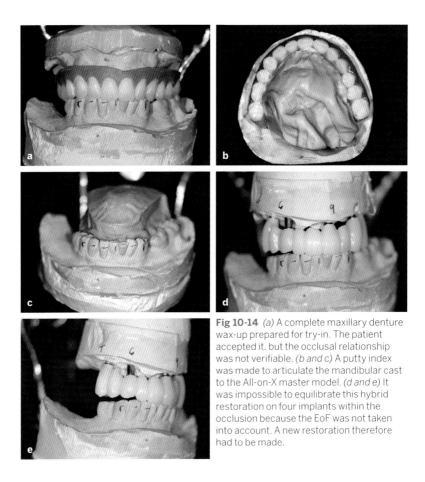

Fig 10-14 *(a)* A complete maxillary denture wax-up prepared for try-in. The patient accepted it, but the occlusal relationship was not verifiable. *(b and c)* A putty index was made to articulate the mandibular cast to the All-on-X master model. *(d and e)* It was impossible to equilibrate this hybrid restoration on four implants within the occlusion because the EoF was not taken into account. A new restoration therefore had to be made.

Recording EoF in Edentulous Cases with Implants

Provisional denture

Similarly to the edentulous cases described above, a trial or provisional denture can be used—with limitations. In cases of immediate loading of the implants with a provisional screw-retained restoration, the options are better. In these clinical situations, we can change or adjust the provisional restoration to the patient's EoF and copy it for the final restoration.

However, due to the difficulty in creating a functional provisional denture, dentists often resort to an approximate one, expecting the laboratory to mimic a good-looking setup of a denture. Figure 10-14 shows

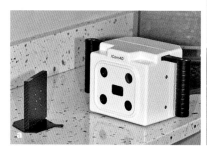

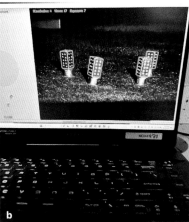

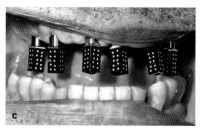

Fig 10-15 *(a to c)* 3D coded abutments placed over implants and precision camera recording the position of the implants to create a digital model.

what this shortcut looks like. In this case, a dentist tried to rush a case of a hybrid restoration on four implants. A wax-up denture was made guided by the existing teeth that needed removal. That setup was transferred with a putty index and related to the edentulous maxillary model (Figs 10-14a to 10-14c). The result was an occlusal relationship far from functional (Figs 10-14d and 10-14e). The prosthesis had to be redone. This is an extreme case of neglecting the interarch registration and the EoF.

Photogrammetry

A more accurate protocol uses implant position cameras and intraoral scanners. Photogrammetry techniques allow a very accurate scan for completely edentulous cases with multiple implant restorations. A high-precision stereo camera (eg, Voxel Dental or PIC Dental) captures the position of 3D coded abutments placed on the implants and creates a very accurate digital model (Fig 10-15). By merging this digital model

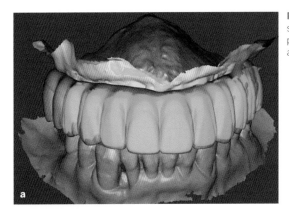

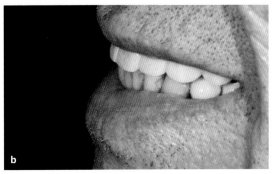

Fig 10-16 *(a and b)* A slightly modified design is produced by widening the arch to improve the EoF.

with an intraoral scan of the existing teeth or analogs, the laboratory can fabricate a polymethyl methacrylate (PMMA) provisional first and a final restoration later. The provisional can be customized intraorally, determining an accurate EoF that can be tested over a period of a few weeks. If needed, the same digital model can be used to create a new and improved provisional, with the esthetics and function approved by the patient (Fig 10-16). When the implants are integrated and the tissue

Customizing the EoF on the prototype restoration and communicating it to the lab has significant benefits: It ensures the patient's satisfaction, minimizes the adjustments needed at the time of delivery of the final restoration, and eliminates the need for major changes that could lead to remaking of the restoration.

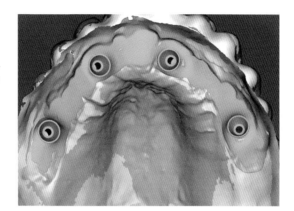

Fig 10-17 The intraoral scan of the intaglio surface is merged with the customized EoF embedded into the provisional scan to fabricate a final restoration.

has healed, a surface intraoral scan of the tissue and of the perfected provisional restoration is taken and merged with the initial implant position scan for fabrication of the final restoration (Fig 10-17).

References

1. The Glossary of Prosthodontic Terms: Ninth Edition. J Prosthet Dent 2017;117(5S):e1–e105.
2. Hoyle DE. Fabrication of a customized anterior guide table. J Prosthet Dent 1982;48:490–491.
3. Tasora A, Simeone P. Development of a new type of incisal table for prosthetic articulators. Int J Dent 2010;2010:458514.

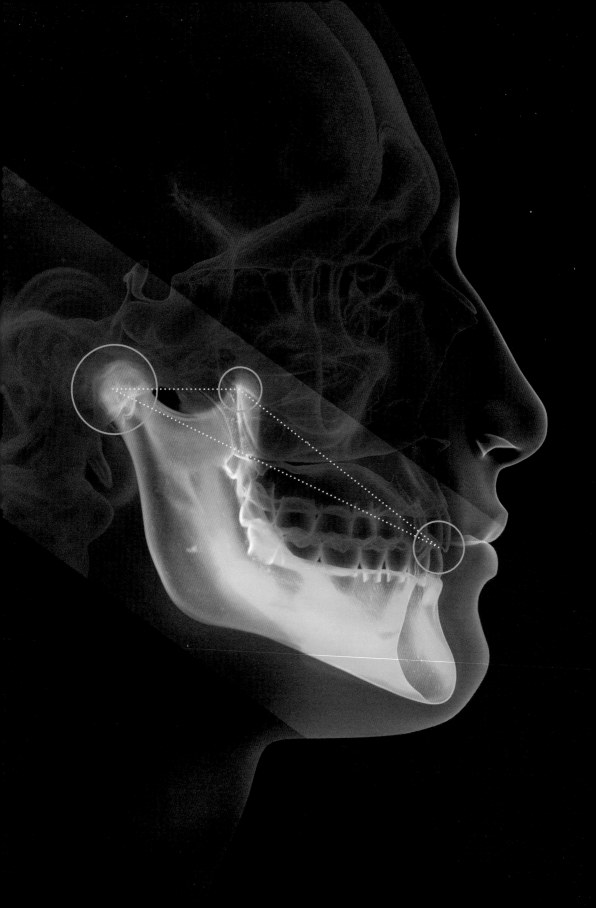

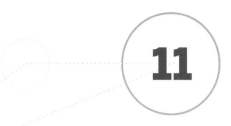

Techniques for Communicating with the Laboratory

With contributions from Lee Culp, CDT

As a young dentist practicing in Germany, I was told that to be a good dentist, all you need is a great technician. Thirty years later, my son Daniel was told that to make good dentures, all you need is a great technician. The dentist-technician relationship is vital to the practice of dentistry.

Lee Culp puts it best: "There is an architect-builder relationship, with the dentist as the architect and the technician as the builder." Builders need a well-designed set of plans, accurate to the site of the building, with precise measurements, clear drawings, a model of the future building, and an overall look to match the expectations of the client. Similarly, dental technicians need accurate impressions or scans of the mouth, clear margins of the preparation, accurate occlusal records, a model of the future restoration in the form of a customized provisional, and the patient's desired shade and other features of the final restoration. Consultations, meetings, and revisions of the plans are common between the architect and the builder. The same must happen between the dentist and the technician. One cannot succeed without the other, and the standards of precision and detail must be fulfilled by both.

The goal of the clinician is to create an accurate virtual patient for the lab to work on. Communication of the occlusal relationship is the most consequential for the final restoration because it is the most difficult to correct when it is missed. The dentist's role is therefore to acquire all clinical data and convey it to the lab, including the following:

- Patient's objectives: desired shape, size, shade
- Dentist's objectives: detailed desired shape, color mapping, texture
- 2D data: photographs of the face and smile, including retracted smile
- 3D data: impressions or scans; interocclusal registrations (static and dynamic); prepreparation models/scans; customized provisionals; jaw-tracking data if available
- Facebow records or digitized facial recordings

The technician's role is to help the dentist design a functional and esthetic prototype and, after the patient's approval, to duplicate it into a final restoration. As part of this process, the technician performs the following tasks:

- Creates a presumptive projection of the future outcome, either an analog or digital diagnostic wax-up, based on the preliminary clinical data; this becomes the 3D blueprint for the patient
- Creates a mock-up in certain cases for the patient to "try in" the restoration before fabrication
- Fabricates provisional restorations using the approved wax-up and mock-up
- Exchanges additional information with the dentist, including impressions, scans, interocclusal registrations, facebow records or facial scans, and/or jaw tracking
- Transfers the clinical data in an analog or virtual articulator
- Copies the functional components customized by the dentist in the patient's mouth into a final restoration that is both functional and esthetic

Fig 11-1 Facebow used to relate the maxillary cast to the articulator.

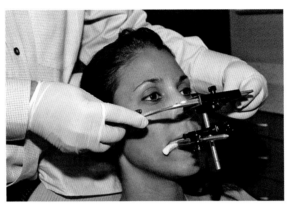

Fig 11-1 Facebow used to relate the maxillary cast to the articulator.

Communication of Occlusion

The desired maxillomandibular relationship in which the technician creates the restoration is the most sensitive piece—and one that is most prone to mistakes. A knowledgeable or gifted technician cannot be a substitute for a sloppy clinical recording. In other words, the lab cannot improve the dentist's imprecise interocclusal registration. While communication with the lab is easier, quicker, and more precise with the digital workflow, the dentist must still capture the bite. If the dentist "misses the bite," the digital data will accurately communicate the inaccuracy to the lab.

Facebow registrations: To use or not to use

The lab needs to create as accurate a simulation of the clinical situation as possible. Historically, the articulator has played an important role in creating such a simulation, especially in relationship to occlusion, and the facebow has served as a key tool in that process (Fig 11-1). The facebow relates the maxillary cast to the hinge axis of the articulator, allows for adjustment of the vertical dimension of occlusion (VDO), and orients the maxillary cast in relation to the occlusal/incisal plane of the patient.

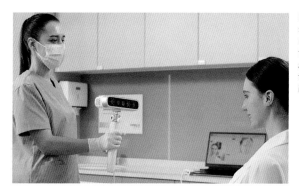

Fig 11-2 A facial scanner captures a 3D image of the patient's face. It can be used as a facebow, relating the face to the digital intraoral scan as well.

However, in the last 15 to 20 years, the role of the facebow has been eroded by the introduction of jaw-tracking devices and facial scanners (Fig 11-2). Jaw-tracking devices (SICAT, Zebris, ModJaw, Theratec) help with the hinge axis and the envelope of function (EoF), and facial scanners (RayFace, Instarisa, Obiscanner, Vectra H2) help determine the incisal plane and, when combined with CBCT imaging, also help with the hinge axis. While it is true that any additional information helps the lab create better, more customized restorations, the question is whether this additional information comes at a reasonable added complexity, time, and financial expense.

The need to find and record the hinge axis for the lab can be circumvented by recording the mandibular position (MP) at the desired VDO. The need to relate the incisal plane to the lab can be achieved with a facial analyzer (Kois) or by using the Bonwill point on a virtual articulator, combined with a facial photograph. The trend is to create precise tools to give the lab an accurate simulation of the patient's masticatory system. Currently, dentists can give the lab sufficient information using the simple tools mentioned above. Let's use those tools we have at our disposal until other ones are perfected and made accessible.

Using an intraoral scan of the customized provisionals is the simplest and most accurate tool to relate the EoF to the lab.

Modalities of Communication

Communication between the dentist and the technician has two components: the data (impressions or scans, occlusal records, facebow records, photography) and personal communication.

The transmission of data ranges from analog to digital. Besides the physical impressions, models, and records,

The analog or digital wax-up is a fundamental piece of communication between the clinician and the lab. It is the architect's set of plans for the builder, approved by the customer.

completely electronic data can also be shared, such as scans, interocclusal registrations, photography, files of jaw movement, and more. In the digital age, the dentist and technician can communicate interactively from across the globe in all phases of the collaboration through teleconferencing software such as Zoom, TeamViewer, GoToMeeting, and more. The architect and the builder can be in constant communication virtually. The patient can also be invited to participate in such communication, adding to the understanding of their objectives, likes, and dislikes.

Communication is a two-way street. The dentist must provide a preliminary plan based on the desired objectives and the occlusion using a reference position at the desired VDO, which allows the technician to project the future restoration in wax or digitally. Changes may need to be made to the first draft, and those must be approved by the patient under the guidance of the dentist. Refinement of the projected restoration and a good plan must be in place before any tooth is touched. New materials, fabrication techniques, and software advancements also allow technicians to more consistently and effectively duplicate the diagnostic wax-ups and customized provisional scans using esthetic materials.

Suggested Protocol

This section details a suggested protocol for a full arch of full-coverage restorations (fixed partial dentures).

Dentist

1. Examination and preliminary treatment planning with the patient
2. Impressions/scans of both arches and photographs
3. Interocclusal registration at the projected MP (centric relation [CR] at the desired VDO)
4. Prescription to the lab for maxillary full-coverage preparation and maintenance of the occlusal plane, with minor adjustments to the mandibular arch, if needed

Technician

5. Fabrication of analog or digital wax-up
6. Mock-up preparation in certain cases

Dentist

7. Patient approval of wax-up and/or mock-up; changes performed if needed

Technician

8. Fabrication of provisional shells or matrices for intraoral fabrication of provisionals

Dentist

9. Preparation of teeth
10. Impressions or scans and interocclusal registrations

Fig 11-3 Photograph with retracted lips to relate the face to the intraoral scans.

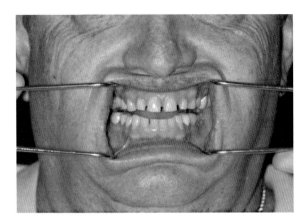

11. Customization of provisionals in closure and excursions and verification of function and esthetics

12. At a subsequent appointment, confirmation of the patient's likes, dislikes, and function, with adjustment as needed

13. Impressions or scans of customized provisionals for the lab

14. Facebow record or facial scan

15. Shade-taking with photography, as well as detailed color mapping with surface texture

16. Photograph of face with retracted lips to make merging of the scans and 2D photograph possible (Fig 11-3).

Technician

17. Creation of the analog or digital patient; the technician now has all the patient's information at their fingertips: face, smile, preparations, opposing model, interocclusal registrations at the desired MP, customized provisionals reproducing the EoF, desired shade, and surface texture

18. Fabrication of the final restoration

Dentist

19. Delivery of the final restoration: Verify and adjust occlusion if needed. Be sure to confirm the patient's acceptance before permanent cementation.

Conclusion

When the clinician thoroughly communicates with the lab, several things happen:

- The technician has complete information and does not need to guess how to fabricate the final restoration.
- The technician works efficiently, eliminating repeated try-ins.
- The dentist saves time by reducing try-ins and minimizing adjustments to the final restorations.
- Patient satisfaction and trust increases.

   The time spent in taking accurate and thorough records and communicating with the lab is well worth the outcome.

As dentists we look only as good as our technician's work, so be sure to use great technicians. On the flip side, a technician's work is reliant on our ability to give them what they need, so always strive to become a better dentist.

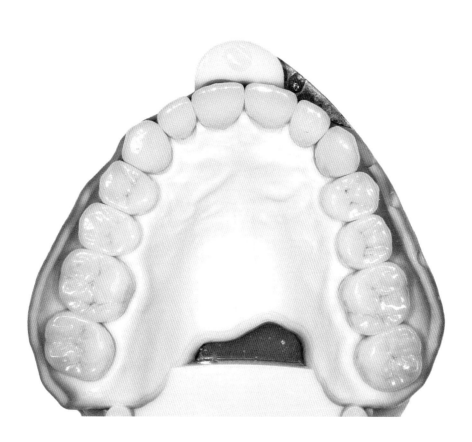

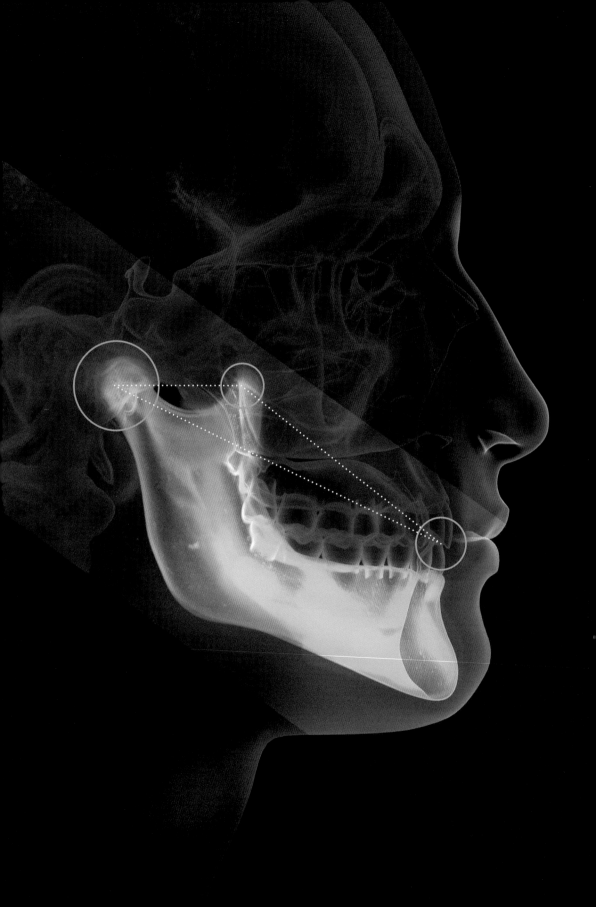

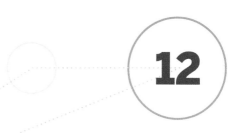

Analog Versus Digital Techniques for Interocclusal Registration

With contributions from Daniel Radu, DMD

Dentistry is changing rapidly from analog to digital, and soon dental workflows will be primarily digital. There are two reasons why we presented both analog and digital workflows in this text: *(1)* Analog workflows are still used by a majority of dentists worldwide; and *(2)* analog protocols are the foundation for digital ones, and some analog tools are still necessary in digital workflows.

Advantages of Digital Workflows

Digital workflows have several advantages over analog workflows (Table 12-1):

- The accuracy of digital intraoral scanners is on par with that of analog impressions, with rare exception (eg, full-arch scanning in edentulous cases with implants).
- The time savings are substantial with the digital workflow, after the initial learning curve is accomplished (see Note I).
- Patient satisfaction, acceptance, and overall experience is improved with the digital workflow.[1,2]

- Transmission of accurate occlusal data to the lab is much more precise with digital workflows.[3–6] The interarch registration does not require a recording medium, such as wax or polyvinyl siloxane, so it is less prone to patient and technician errors.[7,8] This also relieves the technician of the task of mounting the models in the articulator, with all the potential sources of error.
- Digital communication between the clinician and lab is convenient and very precise, which helps in all phases of the restorative process: diagnosis, planning, fabrication of prototypes (provisionals), and transfer of the customized prototypes into the final restoration.

Table 12-1 Comparison of analog and digital workflows		
Analog characteristics	**Digital advantages**	**Digital disadvantages**
Recording medium (wax, polyvinyl siloxane)		
Distortion potential		
Difficulty of evaluation	Easier	
Laboratory mounting potential errors		
Difficult design and fabrication	Easier	
Good accuracy of restorations occlusally	More precise	
Initial equipment investment		Higher
Ease of use and known procedures		Initial learning curve

Conclusion

Labs have adopted digital technologies earlier than clinicians due to the cost savings in design and manufacturing. Many labs digitize the analog records they receive from clinicians and switch to a digital workflow in the lab. While analog protocols are still relevant in clinical practice, digital workflows are the way of the future, so clinicians should investigate the simple and powerful digital tools available to them.

References

1. Giancotti A, Mampieri G, Paoncelli F, Greco M, Arcuri C. Patient's perception of intraoral scanning: A comparison between traditional and digital dental impression. J Biol Regul Homeost Agents 2021;35(3 suppl 1):19–28.
2. Christopoulou I, Kaklamanos EG, Makrygiannakis MA, Bitsanis I, Tsolakis AI. Patient-reported experiences and preferences with intraoral scanners: A systematic review. Eur J Orthod 2022;44:56–65.
3. Revilla-León M, Agustín-Panadero R, Zeitler JM, et al. Differences in maxillo-mandibular relationship recorded at centric relation when using a conventional method, four intraoral scanners, and a jaw tracking system: A clinical study. J Prosthet Dent 2023:S0022-3913(22)00795-8.
4. Morsy N, El Kateb M. Accuracy of intraoral scanners for static virtual articulation: A systematic review and meta-analysis of multiple outcomes. J Prosthet Dent 2022:S0022-3913(22)00608-4.
5. Garikano X, Amezua X, Iturrate M, Solaberrieta E. Evaluation of repeatability of different alignment methods to obtain digital interocclusal records: An in vitro study. J Prosthet Dent 2022:S0022-3913(22)00498-X.
6. Fraile C, Ferreiroa A, Romeo M, Alonso R, Pradíes G. Clinical study comparing the accuracy of interocclusal records, digitally obtained by three different devices. Clin Oral Investig 2022;26:1957–1962.
7. Camci H, Salmanpour F. A new technique for testing accuracy and sensitivity of digital bite registration: A prospective comparative study. Int Orthod 2021;19: 425–432.
8. He M, Ding Q, Li L, et al. The accuracy of transferring casts in maximal intercuspal position to a virtual articulator. J Prosthodont 2022;31:326–332.

Notes

The notes in this section are included to buttress the concepts presented in Parts 1 and 2, bringing some background while reflecting on the current state of the art and looking to the future of dentistry. In this part, we acknowledge the complexity of the subject of occlusion and present uncertainties surrounding this topic. The number(s) in parentheses following each heading indicates the chapter(s) that note supports.

A | The Present State of Occlusion (1)

This text is directed to the restorative dentist. Certain concepts, such as mandibular reference positions, are discussed in depth. Simple physics and other scientific principles help us work toward a new synthesis regarding practical workflows to use in all clinical situations.[1]

In the last 30 years, research has demonstrated that occlusion is not a factor in temporomandibular disease or dysfunction. Arguments range from a lack of conclusive studies proving the relationship to flawed studies showing no correlation to the changing definition of *centric relation* in restorative dentistry.[2]

More recently, emphasis has been placed on the function and position of the tongue in relation to the space and size of the maxilla and mandible. Posterior tongue posture is a prime consideration in airway dentistry, which aims to improve the general health of the patient, not just their teeth.[3]

References

1. Radu M, Marandici M, Hottel TL. The effect of clenching on mandibular position: A vector analysis model. J Prosthet Dent 2004;91:171–179.
2. Kandasamy S, Greene CS, Obrez A. An evidence-based evaluation of the concept of centric relation in the 21st century. Quintessence Int 2018;49:755–760.
3. Coceancig P. 6 Ways to Design a Face: Corrective Jaw Surgery to Optimize Bite, Airway, and Facial Balance. Chicago: Quintessence, 2021.

B | The Terminology of Occlusion (1, 5–8)

"Bad terminology is the enemy of good thinking" – Warren Buffet

The terms we use to explain concepts are not uniform from one dentist to another, and these differing terminologies are responsible for the different "languages" we have for discussing occlusion. Furthermore, as the science of occlusion has evolved, so have our definitions of occlusal concepts, and not everyone is on the same page.

The Glossary of Prosthodontic Terms (GPT) addresses terminology in restorative dentistry in an attempt to set the standard for the field, and the latest version appeared in 2017.[1] Examples of GPT-advocated terminology include occlusion instead of bite, maximal intercuspal position instead of habitual occlusion, fixed partial denture instead of crown, and occlusal device instead of splint or guard. Yet the latter terms—bite, habitual occlusion, crown, and splint/guard—are still used as common lexicon among dentists and their patients. While some dentists are not aware of these terminology changes, others simply disregard them because they think they complicate the issues. This text attempts to thread the needle by using the GPT terminology while trying to simplify and clarify the concepts for the practicing dentist. When helpful, both the official term and the common term are used for explanation of certain concepts. After all, if the terminology gets in the way of understanding, what's the point?

Good terminology has to be descriptive; that is, a term should tell us what it means. The following terms are included to aid understanding throughout the book. A "practical definition" is also provided for each.

Common terms

Occlusion
(O in the occlusion formula)

- *GPT definition:* The static relationship between the incising or masticating surfaces of the maxillary or mandibular teeth or tooth analogs.
- *Practical definition:* The relationship between the maxillary and mandibular teeth.

Intercuspation (IC)

- *GPT definition:* The proximity of cusps of opposing teeth.
- *Practical definition:* How the mandibular teeth contact the maxillary ones.

Maximal intercuspal position (MIP)

- *GPT definition:* The complete intercuspation of the opposing teeth independent of condylar position, sometimes referred to as the best fit of the teeth regardless of the condylar position; synonym: intercuspal position (ICP).
- *Practical definition:* Maximal contact of opposing teeth.
- *Note: MIP is a reference position, and "position" refers to the mandibular position (MP), since that is the only moving part in the system.*

Mandibular position (MP)

- *GPT definition:* Not defined.
- *Practical definition:* The position of the mandible in relation to the maxilla.

Condylar position (CP)

- *GPT definition:* Not defined (but "condylar hinge position" is defined as an obsolete term from the fourth edition of GPT).
- *Practical definition:* The position of the condyles on the articular eminence.
- *Note:* One possible condylar position is centric relation (CR), when condyles are in a fully seated, stable, orthopedically correct position.

Anterior reference point (ARP)

- *GPT definition:* Not defined.
- *Practical definition:* The point at the incisal edge of the mandibular central incisors.
- *Note:* This point can be used as a third point to define the position of the mandible in space, along with the two condylar position points.

162

Vertical dimension of occlusion (VDO)

- *GPT definition:* The distance between two selected anatomical or marked points (usually one on the tip of the nose and the other on the chin) when in maximal intercuspal position.
- *Peter Dawson definition:* The repetitive contracted length of the elevator muscles.
- *Practical definition:* The position of the mandibular incisal point in relation to the maxillary fixed incisors; how far the moving mandible is from the fixed maxilla.
- *Note:* The VDO can be visualized as the mandibular incisal point in space and may be considered as synonymous with the anterior reference point (ARP) when defining the mandibular position.

Centric relation (CR)

- *GPT definition:* A maxillomandibular relationship, independent of tooth contact, in which the condyles articulate in the anterosuperior position against the posterior slopes of the articular eminences; in this position, the mandible is restricted to a purely rotary movement. From this unstrained, physiologic, maxillomandibular relationship, the patient can make vertical, lateral, or protrusive movements. It is a clinically useful, repeatable reference position.
- *Practical definition:* A fully seated, physiologic, orthopedically correct, repeatable, stable condylar position where the elevator muscles naturally place the condyles on the eminences.
- *Note:* The new consensus term is *fully seated condylar position*.[2,3] Nonetheless, *centric relation* is a reference position for the *condyles only*; it does not completely define the mandibular position in space—for that we need to define the position of a third point, the anterior reference point (ARP).

Envelope of function (EoF)

- *GPT definition:* The 3D space contained within the envelope of motion that defines mandibular movement during masticatory function and/or phonation.
- *Practical definition:* The occlusal anatomy harmonious with the mandibular movements in function.
- *Note:* The EoF is the sum trajectory of the mandibular movements while the contacting occlusal surfaces of the mandibular teeth slide on the maxillary teeth.[4,5]

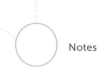
Recording the occlusion

How to record the occlusion for the lab is at the core of this text. There are a whole host of terms used by leaders in the field to refer to that information: *occlusal record*,[6] *interarch relationship*,[7] *intercuspal registration*,[8] *occlusal registration*,[9] *interocclusal record*,[10,11] *bite registration*,[12] and *bite record*.[13] The accepted term in the latest edition of GPT is *interocclusal record* or *maxillomandibular relationship record*. This book uses *interocclusal registration* when describing the techniques of obtaining an interocclusal record.

References

1. Glossary of Prosthodontic Terms, ed 9. J Prosthet Dent 2017;117(5S):e1–e105.
2. Marincel JM. Temporomandibular joint disorders. In: Rosenstiel SF, Lund MF, Walter RD (eds). Contemporary Fixed Prosthodontics. Philadelphia: Elsevier, 2023:122–133.
3. McKee JR. Redefining occlusion. Cranio 2017;35:343–344.
4. Posselt U. Terminal hinge movement of the mandible. 1957. J Prosthet Dent 2001;86:2–9.
5. Nishigawa K, Nakano M, Bando E, Clark GT. Effect of altered occlusal guidance on lateral border movement of the mandible. J Prosthet Dent 1992;68:965–969.
6. Klineberg I, Jagger R (eds). Occlusion and Clinical Practice. Edinburgh: Wright/ Elsevier, 2004:61.
7. Wiskott A. Fixed Prosthodontics: Principles and Clinics. Berlin: Quintessence, 2011:582.
8. Wassell R, Naru A, Steele J. Applied Occlusion. London: Quintessence, 2008.
9. Fradeani M, Barducci G. Esthetic Rehabilitation in Fixed Prosthodontics, Vol 2: Prosthetic Treatment. Milan: Quintessence, 2008.
10. Shillingburg HT Jr, Sather DA, Wilson EL Jr, et al. Fundamentals of Fixed Prosthodontics, ed 4. Chicago: Quintessence, 2012.
11. Okeson JP. Management of Temporomandibular Disorders and Occlusion, ed 8. St Louis: Mosby, 2019.
12. Spear FM. Fundamental occlusal therapy considerations. In: McNeill C (ed). Science and Practice of Occlusion. Chicago: Quintessence, 1997:421–434.
13. Dawson PE. Functional Occlusion: From TMJ to Smile Design. St Louis: Mosby, 2006.

C | To Keep or Change the Existing Occlusion (6)

Many clinical situations allow treatment in the existing occlusion, yet there are plenty of clinical situations when the occlusion is missing or it must be altered to obtain restorative space[1] or resolve occlusal muscle problems. Whether to keep or change the occlusion is in reality a treatment planning decision. The questions we need to answer are the following:

- **Can we safely open the vertical dimension of occlusion (VDO) for restorative purposes?** Some dentists believe that if the intercuspation is changed "just a little," they are effectively keeping the old intercuspation, but that is simply not true. When we change the intercuspation, we lose whatever was there. There is also a belief among dentists that we should always keep the existing occlusion because we don't know what will happen if we change it. That is also a flawed supposition. The truth is that the VDO can be opened safely, such as in wear cases, if we create a new stable mandibular position in the fully seated condylar position. In other words, if the opening is kept within the natural limits of condylar movement (ie, not translating the condyles down the eminence), we can open the VDO, sometimes by as much as 4 to 6 mm anteriorly.

- **How should we open the bite?** A better question is how do we get a stable mandibular position if we modify the existing bite. The answer: A stable mandibular position has a stable condylar position and anterior reference point. Besides the stability in the static occlusion, we also need to customize the envelope of function of the new restoration.

- **Should we change the occlusion to address occlusal muscle problems?** This is a controversial topic.[2–4] Multiple aspects of dentistry must be considered, such as the cause-effect relationship, adaptability of systems, philosophies of occlusion, ethics of human studies, and difficulties in obtaining evidence-based research. Did the occlusion cause the patient's problem? The literature supports both "Yes" and "No" answers.[2–4] But if we cannot agree that occlusion has caused the problem, then we cannot agree that a change is needed.

  My suggestion is to take a practical approach: evaluate, inform, recommend, and act if needed:
  – Evaluate all structures involved in the occlusion in all cases.
  – Present the findings to the patient.
  – If there are signs and symptoms of instability, make recommendations regarding altering the occlusion. One way to temporarily alter the occlusion and achieve a stable mandibular position is with occlusal devices. Like a test drive, we can verify our hypothesis that changing the occlusion will resolve the symptoms or not.

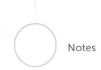

– If a change in occlusion is needed to fulfill the restorative or esthetic needs, use the least invasive treatment modalities to reestablish a new occlusion.

I do not advocate changing all "imperfect" (ie, unstable) occlusions to prevent future problems. Instead, evaluate periodically to see whether eventual changes warrant an intervention. This approach takes into account the adaptability of each individual patient.

• **Is a change in occlusion predictable?** Stability is the reason an existing occlusion, or a given intercuspation, is comfortable to the patient and is safe to use when possible. When changing the occlusion, we have to stabilize the mandible orthopedically by finding a stable condylar position at the desired VDO and recreate the intercuspation in that position. The new intercuspation will further stabilize the mandible and create comfort immediately.

References

1. Spear FM. Occlusal consideration for complex restorative therapy. In: McNeill C (ed). Science and Practice of Occlusion. Chicago: Quintessence, Chicago, 1997:437–456.
2. Safari A, Jowkar Z, Farzin M. Evaluation of the relationship between bruxism and premature occlusal contacts. J Contemp Dent Pract 2013;14:616–621.
3. Clark GT, Tsukiyama Y, Baba K, Watanabe T. Sixty-eight years of experimental occlusal interference studies: What have we learned? J Prosthet Dent 1999;82:704–713.
4. Gher ME. Changing concepts. The effects of occlusion on periodontitis. Dent Clin North Am 1998;42:285–299.

D | Stability and Adaptability of the Stomatognathic System (2, 8, 9)

Stability and adaptability are general properties of systems. Like any natural system, the stomatognathic system seeks stability, but it exhibits adaptability as well. These two seem complementary to each other: changes in stability are corrected by adaptation processes.

The human body is very adaptable. Our skin gets tough and grows calluses with use, our muscles grow in response to repeated application of force, and our eyes dilate and constrict based on how much light is available. But a sharp object will pierce even the most calloused skin, even professional weightlifters cannot lift more than their muscle mass allows, and a sudden flash of light will always blind us momentarily.

Even in states of disease, the body still adapts. In the case of slow artery blockage through plaque accumulation, the collateral circulation will compensate up to a certain point. But in a sudden blockage event, such as an embolus, there is no time for the system to adapt, and serious consequences will always follow (ie, stroke or heart attack). The body needs time to adapt; otherwise, it cannot make the necessary compensations.

Similarly, in our stomatognathic system, teeth erupt and settle in occlusion over the course of many years. The adaptation process, in the form of tooth migration or wear and muscle, bone, and joint remodeling, has time to produce stability at the level of intercuspation. If we suddenly change the intercuspation, for example in restorative cases, the adaptive processes do not have the time to compensate through remodeling, and patients may experience symptoms of discomfort, pain, or breakage of restorations. In full-arch restorative dentistry, *stability* must be a prime goal, not the hope for adaptability to compensate for flaws in the construction.

Stability

In terms of the occlusion formula, we may consider the stability of intercuspation (IC) or mandibular position (MP) or both. A stability limited to IC is sufficient in many individuals. Complete stability may be obtained through a harmony between the IC, joints, and muscles (musculoskeletally stable joints).[1,2]

Complete stability is not a prerequisite for optimal function of the system. We cannot and should not impose norms of stability to all masticatory systems. At the same time, however, lack of stability in a system should not be discounted or rejected as a potential contributing factor in the development of signs or symptoms and therefore neglected in our treatments.[3–5] **The principle of stability should govern our treatments and techniques for interocclusal registration** (see chapter 2).

A majority of individuals have stability provided by a stable maximal intercuspal position acquired over time through various adaptative processes. That stable occlusion should be recorded for the lab when we treat in the existing occlusion (see chapter 7). When we create a new occlusion for our treatment, we need to find a stable MP to work in. Fully seated

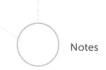
condyles at the desired vertical dimension of occlusion (VDO) create that stable MP, which should be recorded for the lab (see chapter 8).

The rules for stability are as follows:

- Stability limited to intercuspation:
  - Stable stops on all teeth
  - Disocclusion of all posterior teeth in all movements
- Complete stability[1]:
  - Stable stops on all teeth when the condyles are fully seated
  - Disocclusion of all posterior teeth in all movements
  - Anterior guidance in harmony with the envelope of function

Adaptability

Adaptability of living systems involves changes to their internal states in response to changes in their environments to ensure their survival and fitness.[6]

The adaptability of the stomatognathic system is well documented in the literature.[7–11] In orthodontics, it can be difficult to achieve a stable mandible during treatment. The "settling" of teeth into the occlusion after treatment completion is an example of adaptability: teeth move slightly to adapt to the forces exerted upon them.[12] But there are also studies showing the opposite, that after orthodontic treatment, the occlusal contacts do not improve spontaneously.[13,14]

Some authors suggest that finding a stable condylar position for treatment is not necessary because the condyles will adapt to a new intercuspation.[15] But in restorative dentistry we should not have to rely on adaptability to create stability over time. When we create a new occlusion, we can achieve stability by placing the condyles and the anterior reference point in stable positions to create a new harmonious intercuspation. That achieves immediate stability.

While adaptability seems to be a friend, it may actually be an enemy of stability if it offers us an excuse for not taking all the necessary steps to ensure stability through our therapies. Adaptability is a help—not a substitute—for stability. We should not start from the premise that adaptability is going to prevail over any instability we may introduce into the system. **We should strive for stability to reduce the need for adaptability.**

References

1. Dawson PE. Functional Occlusion: From TMJ to Smile Design. St Louis: Mosby, 2006.
2. Pokorny PH, Wiens JP, Litvak H. Occlusion for fixed prosthodontics: A historical perspective of the gnathological influence. J Prosthet Dent 2008;99:299–313.
3. Zonnenberg AJJ. A Data-Supported Reference Position of the Intermaxillary Relationship [dissertation]. Utrecht, The Netherlands: Utrecht University, 2014.
4. Peck CC. Biomechanics of occlusion—Implications for oral rehabilitation. J Oral Rehabil 2016;43:205–214.
5. Spear FM. Fundamental occlusal therapy considerations. In: McNeill C (ed). Science and Practice of Occlusion. Chicago: Quintessence, 1997:421–434.
6. Tu Y, Rappel WJ. Adaptation of living systems. Annu Rev Condens Matter Phys 2018;9:183–205.
7. Voudouris JC, Kuftinec MM. Improved clinical use of Twin-block and Herbst as a result of radiating viscoelastic tissue forces on the condyle and fossa in treatment and long-term retention: Growth relativity. Am J Orthod Dentofacial Orthop 2000;117:247–266.
8. Okeson JP. Evolution of occlusion and temporomandibular disorder in orthodontics: Past, present, and future. Am J Orthod Dentofacial Orthop 2015;147(5 suppl):S216–S223.
9. Woda A, Pionchon P, Palla S. Regulation of mandibular postures: Mechanisms and clinical implications. Crit Rev Oral Biol Med 2001;12:166–178.
10. Wiens JP, Priebe JW. Occlusal stability. Dent Clin North Am 2014;58:19–43.
11. Hellmann D, Glöggler JC, Plaschke K, et al. Effects of preventing intercuspation on the precision of jaw movements. J Oral Rehabil 2021;48:392–402.
12. Littlewood SJ, Millett DT, Doubleday B, Bearn DR, Worthington HV. Retention procedures for stabilising tooth position after treatment with orthodontic braces. Cochrane Database Syst Rev 2004;(1):CD002283.
13. Morton S, Pancherz H. Changes in functional occlusion during the postorthodontic retention period: A prospective longitudinal clinical study. Am J Orthod Dentofacial Orthop 2009;135:310–315.
14. Cohen-Lévy J, Boulos C, Rompré P, Montpetit A, Kerstein RB. Is the quality of occlusal contacts comparable after aligner and fixed orthodontic therapy? A non-randomized cohort comparison using computerized occlusal analysis during 6 months of retention [epub ahead of print 1 April 2022]. Cranio doi: 10.1080/08869634.2022.2056688.
15. Kandasamy S, Greene CS, Obrez A. An evidence-based evaluation of the concept of centric relation in the 21st century. Quintessence Int 2018;49:755–760.

E | Why We Need Centric Relation (Fully Seated Condylar Position) in Restorative Dentistry (6, 8)

Chapter 8 describes how to perform an interocclusal registration for a new occlusion in various clinical situations, emphasizing the common denominators and practical techniques to use when we need to create a new occlusion. This Note is about *why* we do it that way.

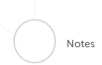

When the maximal intercuspal position (MIP) is missing, we need another reference position. McNeill[1] suggests myocentric or centric relation (CR) in such cases. The myocentric position has the mandible in a rest position obtained by electric stimulation (TENSE),[2] where the condyles are not seated on the eminences. It is not a functional position and difficult to record, so it is not recommended. CR reference position has the condyles seated in a functional, musculoskeletally stable position on the eminences.[3] It is a stable, repeatable position under load, which is why it is recommended for use in all the clinical situations presented in chapter 8.

To bring clarity to this topic, we will first discuss why centric relation is controversial and then learn why it is still the most reasonable reference position to adopt when the intercuspation is missing.

> **The real debate about CR is how to define it, how to find it, and when to use it.**

Why is CR controversial?

The term *centric relation* is semantically objectionable.[4] Research has shown that the condyles are not in the center of the fossae, so the term is not quite accurate. The concept also describes only the condylar position, not the mandibular position, which we need to determine and record. CR was first introduced in the 1920s and has been redefined about every 10 years. Over the course of its evolution, *centric relation* has come to mean many different things: the most retruded position of the mandible; the midmost, uppermost position of the mandible to the maxilla; and the anterosuperior position of the condyles in the fossae.

Originally CR was introduced for fully edentulous cases[6] and later recommended for all clinical situations. Some authors saw CR as the gold standard of occlusion,[7] from single-tooth restorations to orthodontic treatment and management of temporomandibular disorders (TMDs). Most rejections of CR as the standard for treatment comes from ortho-dontic[8] and TMD[9] studies.

Fig 1 A ball in a bowl travels under the force of gravity down the wall until it reaches the bottom, where the translation force is zero.

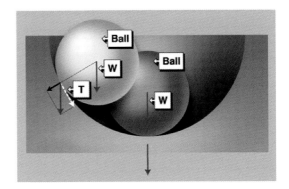

Fig 2 The condyle in the fossa (upside down in this image) is like a ball in a bowl.

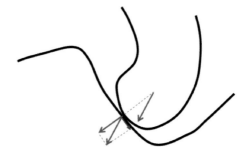

Why is CR a reasonable reference position to use when the intercuspation is missing?

There is a movement growing to change or abandon the very name CR.[4] Some authors propose the term *musculoskeletally stable position*,[10] and the term *fully seated condylar position*[11,12] has lately been embraced as a descriptive definition of CR. Today CR should be defined as a fully seated condylar position, which is why we used these concepts interchangeably in the text. The consensus appears to be that CR should be used in cases where we need a stable, reproducible jaw position other than the MIP.[4,9] Restorative dentistry includes many situations with missing intercuspation or the need to change the existing intercuspation. In those cases, CR is the reference mandibular position of choice.[5,13]

A useful analogy for the condyle in the fossa is to consider a ball in a bowl. In function under the load of the elevator muscles, the condyles naturally reach the fully seated position, just like a ball naturally travels to the bottom of a bowl due to the force of gravity, eventually stopping when the translation force equals zero (Figs 1 and 2).

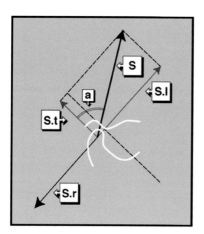

Fig 3 The trigonometry of CR.

Similarly, in the absence of the translation force, the condyle won't move. In other words, the condyle is stable when the forces applied to it are perpendicular to the articular eminence (fossa). For the other math lovers out there, Fig 3 explains the trigonometry at work here. Using the formula $S.t = S*cos\ a$, when the angle a is 90 degrees, the translation force is zero. I delved into the math after Peter Dawson challenged me to demonstrate mathematically why CR is a reference position of choice.[14]

The patient's elevator muscles, with relaxed lateral pterygoids, determine the position of the condyles in the articular fossae, not the clinician's hands. The clinician has to create the anterior obstacle to allow the mandible to slide, instruct the patient to move the mandible back and forth, and make sure that the same position is acquired repeatedly.

The origin and insertion of the muscles will vary from patient to patient. Therefore, the condylar position (and the CR) becomes very individualized. Bimanual manipulation may not be able to achieve that. This representation may explain why CR is potentially not one spot, but an area or zone, as some publications advocate.[15,16] This also may explain the "long centric" concept. The vector force of the elevator muscles may be different in the supine than the upright position, based on the variation in recruitment of muscle fibers.

This anatomical and geometric study validates the techniques using an anterior obstacle to find a stable condylar position, such as a leaf gauge, Lucia jig, composite resin jig, or gothic arch device.

References

1. McNeill C. Fundamental treatment goals. In: McNeill C (ed). Science and Practice of Occlusion. Chicago: Quintessence, 1997:309–311.
2. Jankelson B. Neuromuscular Dental Diagnosis and Treatment. St Louis: Ishiaku EuroAmerica, 1990.
3. Okeson JP, Kazumi I. Orthodontic therapy and the temporomandibular disorder patient. In: Graber LW, Vanarsdall RL, Vig KWL (eds). Orthodontics: Current Principles and Techniques, ed 5. St Louis: Mosby, 2012:179–192.
4. Zonnenberg AJJ, Türp JC, Greene CS. Centric relation critically revisited—What are the clinical implications? J Oral Rehabil 2021;48:1050–1055.
5. Becker CM, Kaiser DA, Schwalm C. Mandibular centricity: Centric relation. J Prosthet Dent 2000;83:158–160.
6. Hanau RL. Articulation defined, analyzed and formulated. J Am Dent Assoc 1926;13:1694–1709.
7. Dawson PE. Functional Occlusion: From TMJ to Smile Design. St Louis: Mosby, 2006.
8. Kandasamy S, Greene CS. The evolution of temporomandibular disorders: A shift from experience to evidence. J Oral Pathol Med 2020;49:461–469.
9. Kandasamy S, Greene CS, Obrez A. An evidence-based evaluation of the concept of centric relation in the 21st century. Quintessence Int 2018;49:755–760.
10. Okeson JP. Evolution of occlusion and temporomandibular disorder in orthodontics: Past, present, and future. Am J Orthod Dentofacial Orthop 2015;147(5 suppl):S216–S223.
11. Marincel JM. Temporomandibular joint disorders. In: Rosenstiel SF, Lund MF, Walter RD (eds). Contemporary Fixed Prosthodontics. Philadelphia: Elsevier, 2023:122–133.
12. McKee JR. Redefining occlusion. Cranio 2017;35:343–344.
13. Radu M, Radu D, Abboud M. Digital recording of a conventionally determined centric relation: A technique using an intraoral scanner. J Prosthet Dent 2020;123:228–231.
14. Radu M, Marandici M, Hottel T. The effect of clenching on condylar position: A vector analysis model. J Prosthet Dent 2004;91:171–179.
15. Celenza FV. The theory and clinical management of centric positions: II. Centric relation and centric relation occlusion. Int J Periodontics Restorative Dent 1984;4:62–86.
16. Wiens JP, Goldstein GR, Andrawis M, Choi M, Priebe JW. Defining centric relation. J Prosthet Dent 2018;120:114–122.

F | Complex Cases and TMJ Problems (6, 8)

Jaw joint problems need to be diagnosed and addressed in the process of treating the dentition. Therefore, a general dentist must have a core knowledge of the temporomandibular joint (TMJ) and know how to manage patients with such problems. The screening examination has to uncover potential jaw joint problems, a diagnosis has to be made, and a course of action needs to be established (see chapter 6).

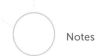

Some occlusal philosophies contend that occlusion may cause sore muscles and dysfunctional joints.[1-4] The assumption is that microtrauma to the disc, produced by the constant contraction of the lateral pterygoid muscles, causes most cases of temporomandibular disorder (TMD). More recently, the pendulum has swung to the contention that occlusion has nothing to do with TMD.[5,6] Instead, it is believed that a macrotrauma to the joint, many times undiagnosed, is often the cause of the disc injury and subsequent TMD. Occlusion may be only a contributing factor, not a cause of the problem. Investigating the joints using MRI and CBCT may show a higher than expected internal derangement of the joints.[7] If the growth center of the condyle is not protected by the disc during the growth phase of the individual, the condyle and ramus have significant deficiencies, with occlusal and facial consequences.[8,9]

In addition to macrotrauma, there are several medical conditions affecting the head and neck that may also be responsible for symptoms and dysfunction: cluster headaches, migraine, reflex sympathetic dystrophy, fibromyalgia, and more. Because of these multiple potential causes of problems in the stomatognathic system, orofacial pain is now recognized as the 12th dental specialty by the American Dental Association.

In the field of occlusion and TMD, one can find literature supporting the relation between the two[10,11] and also rejecting it.[12,13] Some authors suggest that the mechanistic model of occlusion, in which a "ridged" condylar position is prescribed, should be replaced by a "medical model" of occlusion.[12,14] In this medical model, all possible factors may play a role in the symptomatology of TMD, with the exception of the condylar position.[15]

It is difficult for the practicing dentist to sift through the literature and form an opinion, especially when it comes to applying the latest research in daily practice. Indeed, a practicing dentist has several options: diagnose and inform the patient; treat the patient for the jaw joint issues as well as the other concerns; or refer the patient for the TMD and treat later. First and foremost, all dentists must possess a core knowledge in the field of TMD and occlusion; that is the prerequisite for a diagnosis, which is the cornerstone of the therapeutic approach. Based on the level of expertise and experience, some clinical situations may be treated by the diagnosing clinician, and some may need to be referred. The referral should be based on the diagnosis and may be to one or multiple clinicians:

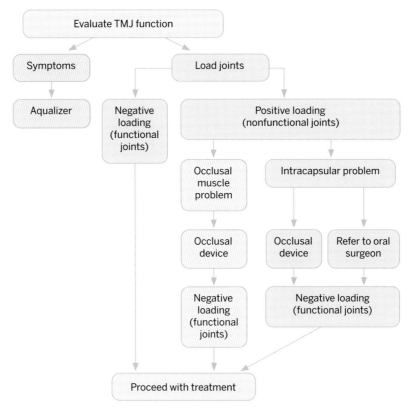

Fig 1 Clinical guideline for treating patients with TMJ problems.

TMD/orofacial pain specialist; ear, nose, and throat specialist; maxillofacial surgeon; neurologist; chiropractor; or physical therapist.

This text addresses what a dentist with a solid knowledge of the TMJ can do to treat patients with TMD. Restorative work should be performed only *after* resolving the jaw joint conditions. Specific textbooks, courses, residencies, and specialties are recommended resources before treating patients with such problems.[15–17]

The clinical guideline below helps the dentist make treatment decisions (Fig 1).

1. **Diagnose the problem:** If the TMJs reveal pain or discomfort upon loading, it means they cannot properly function. Any restorative treatment should be postponed until the resolution of the jaw symptoms. The pain upon loading may be from two sources: muscle pain or joint pain (intracapsular). The muscles that exhibit pain upon loading are mainly the lateral pterygoid muscles (when they are stretched by the bimanual manipulation) or the elevator muscles (from the patient clenching). The intracapsular pain may be from the condyles compressing the retrodiscal attachment when the disc is displaced anteriorly or from a damaged bone structure (osteoarthritis).

2. **Treat the muscles/joints before any restorative work:** A stabilizing occlusal device is a simple and effective way to relax the muscles and heal the joints.[18,19] It is recommended that the patient wear the occlusal device for 8 to 12 weeks, with weekly adjustments, or until complete resolution of the symptoms. The patient should wear the device every night during sleep and preferably more throughout the day, not to exceed 12 hours daily[20]; it can even be worn while chewing if possible. 3D imaging is helpful to determine the prognosis and make the patient aware of future possible changes and needed adjustments.

3. **Maintain the stable mandibular position:** Only when the patient is pain free upon loading should a restorative treatment be performed. It is critical to create a new intercuspation in harmony with the stable, fully seated condylar position. That will ensure the stability of the mandible and of the stomatognathic system and minimize the occurrence of future occlusal-induced muscle problems. That may include one or more of the following treatment modalities: equilibration, orthodontics, restorative therapy, and orthognathic surgery.

4. **Enroll the patient in a long-term maintenance program:** It is recommended to equilibrate the final restoration and check it periodically for possible bony remodeling, which will require refinement of the occlusion. A protective occlusal device should also be given to the patient. A hard CR device, adjusted periodically, is recommended. A soft device, such as a vacuum-formed one, may introduce occlusal interferences and is not recommended (see note on occlusal devices). Even advanced cases with condylar resorption may be handled with occlusal devices until the resolution of the symptoms.

References

1. Dawson PE. Position paper regarding diagnosis, management, and treatment of temporomandibular disorders. J Prosthet Dent 1999;81:174.
2. Solow RA. The dental literature on occlusion and myogenous orofacial pain: Application of critical thinking. Cranio 2016;34:323–331.
3. Cordray FE. The relationship between occlusion and TMD. Open J Stomatol 2017;7.
4. Mitchell RJ. Etiology of temporomandibular disorders. Curr Opin Dent 1991;1:471.
5. Gremillion HA. The relationship between occlusion and TMD: An evidence-based discussion. J Evid Based Dent Pract 2006;6:43–47.
6. Kalladka M, Young A, Thomas D, Heir GM, Quek SYP, Khan J. The relation of temporomandibular disorders and dental occlusion: A narrative review. Quintessence Int 2022;53:450–459.
7. Valesan LF, Doebber Da-Cas C, Réus JC, et al. Prevalence of temporo-mandibular joint disorders: A systematic review and meta-analysis. Clin Oral Investig 2021;25:441–453.
8. Pressman BD. MR imaging of temporomandibular joint abnormalities associated with cervical hyperextension/hyperflexion (whiplash) injuries. J Magn Reson Imaging 1992;2:569–574.
9. Flores-Mir C. Longitudinal study of temporomandibular joint disc status and craniofacial growth. Am J Orthod Dentofacial Orthop 2006;130:324–330.
10. Okeson JP, Kazumi I. Orthodontic therapy and the temporomandibular disorder patient. In: Graber LW, Vanarsdall RL, Vig KWL (eds). Orthodontics: Current Principles and Techniques, ed 5. St Louis: Mosby, 2012:179–192.
11. Roth HR. Gnathologic considerations for orthodontic therapy. In: McNeill (ed). Science and Practice of Occlusion. Chicago: Quintessence, 1997:502–512.
12. Kandasamy S, Greene CS. The evolution of temporomandibular disorders: A shift from experience to evidence. J Oral Pathol Med 2020;49:461–469.
13. Greene CS, Manfredini D. Transitioning to chronic temporomandibular disorder pain: A combination of patient vulnerabilities and iatrogenesis. J Oral Rehabil 2021;48:1077–1088.
14. Greene CS, Manfredini D. Treating temporomandibular disorders in the 21st century: Can we finally eliminate the "third pathway"? J Oral Facial Pain Headache 2020;34:206–216.
15. Kandasamy S, Greene CS, Obrez A. An evidence-based evaluation of the concept of centric relation in the 21st century. Quintessence Int 2018;49:755–760.
16. Okeson JP. Management of Temporomandibular Disorders and Occlusion, ed 8. St Louis: Mosby, 2019.
17. Marincel JM. Temporomandibular joint disorders. In: Rosenstiel SF, Lund MF, Walter RD (eds). Contemporary Fixed Prosthodontics. Philadelphia: Elsevier, 2023:122–133.
18. Alkhutari AS, Alyahya A, Rodrigues Conti PC, Christidis N, Al-Moraissi EA. Is the therapeutic effect of occlusal stabilization appliances more than just placebo effect in the management of painful temporomandibular disorders? A network meta-analysis of randomized clinical trials. J Prosthet Dent 2021;126:24–32.
19. Fricton J, Look JO, Wright E, et al. Systematic review and meta-analysis of randomized controlled trials evaluating intraoral orthopedic appliances for temporomandibular disorders. J Orofac Pain 2010;24:237–254.
20. Lee CF, Proffit WR. The daily rhythm of tooth eruption. Am J Orthod Dentofacial Orthop 1995;107:38–47.

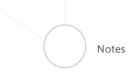

G | Rationale for Occlusal Devices (8)

The goal of any device inserted in between the teeth is to change the existing intercuspation, and therefore the mandibular position, because we consider it nonphysiologic. Occlusal muscles problems may also be addressed using such devices.[1] We may want to create a new occlusal scheme and test it, redirect the forces of the masticatory muscles, or protect the teeth or restorations from excessive forces.

The centric relation splint is a permissive splint in that it allows the mandible to move freely and find a physiologic, orthopedically correct, stable position. It may be considered a dry run for more permanent occlusal interventions, such as restorative or orthodontic procedures. These splints are widely used with well-documented positive results.[2,3]

An occlusal device is a simple way for a dentist to work and experience the geometry of the occlusion. It is a way to practice reversable occlusal therapy. It is a test drive to determine if the mandibular position combined with the existing intercuspation caused the patient's symptoms. The occlusal device is a temporary occlusal therapy, followed by a permanent one, such as equilibration, restorations, or orthodontics. Some patients may elect to forgo permanent therapy and use the occlusal device for an extended period of time with satisfactory results.

The controversy mentioned in Note F is also found in the use of occlusal devices. Some studies suggest that clinicians should reconsider the paradigm relating prematurities in centric relation and slides to temporomandibular disorders.[4]

It is important to note that not all devices are created equal. Devices should never by fabricated by arbitrarily opening the vertical dimension of occlusion on an articulator, and over-the-counter devices cannot be customized and adjusted to a physiologic mandibular position.

References

1. Solow RA. Customized anterior guidance for occlusal devices: Classification and rationale. J Prosthet Dent 2013;110:259–263.
2. Fleigel JD 3rd, Sutton AJ. Reliable and repeatable centric relation adjustment of the maxillary occlusal device. J Prosthodont 2013;22:233–236.
3. Kidder GM, Solow RA. Precision occlusal splints and the diagnosis of occlusal problems in myogenous orofacial pain patients. Gen Dent 2014;62:24–31.
4. Manfredini D. Temporomandibular disorders and dental occlusion. A systematic review of association studies: End of an era? J Oral Rehabil 2017;11:908–923.

H | Classifications of Occlusion (6)

A classification of occlusion helps us understand the system and communicate with our patients and fellow clinicians. Classifications should not only be accurate but also should be useful in making clinical decisions.

The two major classifications in occlusion are Angle's classification of malocclusion, used predominantly in orthodontics, and Dawson's classification of occlusion. Angle's classification is a tool used to visualize the relationship of the mandible to the maxilla, evaluating the interdigitation of the arches. The condylar position and anterior reference point position are not taken into account. While this method can be considered a classification of intercuspation, it is an incomplete representation of the occlusal system.

Dawson's classification of occlusion[1,2] is based on the relationship between maximal intercuspal position and the position and condition of the temporomandibular joints (TMJs). It takes into account both intercuspation and mandibular position, and it also considers the condition of the joints, which is relevant to the function and stability of the system. It is a useful classification for clinical applications because it guides the clinician to accept or change the mandibular position before proceeding with treatment. The difficulty comes in evaluating the condition of the joints, for example in discerning if the disc is properly aligned with the condyle. We may need imaging to determine the condition of the condyles. Because of this difficulty, I propose a simplified classification of occlusion from a clinical, practical perspective, based on function and stability.

When the TMJs accept loading bimanually or while clenching on an anterior obstacle, it means the joints are functional. Therefore, these occlusions can be classified as functional. Joints may be functional if they have a slide or not. When we need to create a new occlusion, the most important consideration is to fully seat the condyles in a physiologic, orthopedically correct position.

TMJs that cannot accept loading without discomfort or pain are nonfunctional. It is important to know if the cause is an occlusal muscle problem, an acute joint problem, or a chronic progressive disorder. The clinical approach is to resolve the problem before we proceed with treatment.

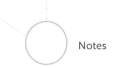

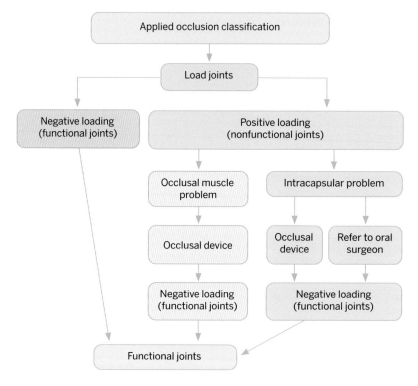

Fig 1 Guideline on how to apply the simplified occlusion classification.

This simplified classification of occlusion as functional or nonfunctional is practical. It is a red or green light to treatment (Fig 1).

Only about 1% of patients in a general practice have unstable joints that cannot accept loading after proper occlusal device therapy. Those patients must be referred to oral surgeons before any permanent change in occlusion is made. That being said, just because few patients present with these problems does not mean that we can get by with little knowledge of the TMJs and occlusion. Knowledge is power—power to diagnose and help our patients to the best of our ability.

References

1. Dawson PE. New definitions for relating occlusion to varying conditions of the temporomandibular joint. J Prosthet Dent 1996;75:619–627.
2. Dawson PE. A classification system for occlusions that relates maximal intercuspation to the position and condition of the temporomandibular joint. J Prosthet Dent 1996;75:60–66.

▌▎ The Economics of Occlusion (12)

In restorative dentistry, an important variable is the time needed to achieve the desired result. In other words, we want the restorations to fit well in the first attempt. Aside from the impressions or scans, the interocclusal registrations are critical to the time spent to fit the restorations.

This book offers a simple, predictable, and basically free way to get precise interocclusal registrations in all clinical situations, especially in those potentially prone to mistakes. If you follow the protocols, you will save a lot of time with no added cost.

The protocols cost nothing to use and take less time than that required for lengthy adjustments, sending work back to the lab for another try-in, or remaking it. The analog workflows require no special equipment or time spent learning how to use it. While the digital workflows do require an equipment and time investment, the benefits are significant (see chapter 12).

For all practicing dentists, time is money, and protocols are the best way to save that money. I've recorded the time spent using and not using protocols and performed an in-depth analysis of analog vs digital workflows for all clinical procedures (interocclusal, envelope of function recordings, fitting of restorations, occlusal adjustments). While these calculations are on file, my summary is as follows:

- Digital workflows are about 50% shorter than analog ones.
- Any time savings are lost when not following a consistent protocol.
- Using protocols saves about 50% of time in analog workflows and 70% of time in digital workflows.

Using protocols saves time and money, and this text is a plea to follow protocols for your interocclusal registrations.

> **If I had to distill this book into one phrase, it would be this: Because we cannot easily measure if our interocclusal registrations are precise, we must follow protocols to ensure accuracy of the records and therefore treatment success.**

Index